History of Medieval Medicine

Contents

Chapter 1

Introduction

1.1 Medieval medicine of Western Europe

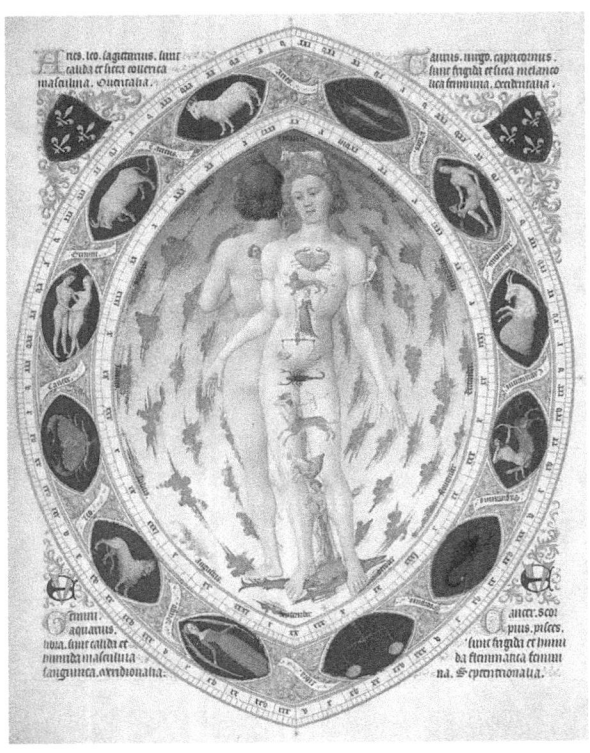

"Anatomical Man" (also "Zodiacal Man"), Très Riches Heures du Duc de Berry *(Ms.65, f.14v, early 15th century)*

Medieval medicine in Western Europe was composed of a mixture of existing ideas from antiquity, spiritual influences and what Claude Lévi-Strauss identifies as the "shamanistic complex" and "social consensus."[1]

In the Early Middle Ages, following the fall of the Western Roman Empire, standard medical knowledge was based chiefly upon surviving Greek and Roman texts, preserved in monasteries and elsewhere. Many simply placed their hopes in the church and God to heal all their sicknesses.

Ideas about the origin and cure of disease were not purely secular, but were also based on a world view in which factors such as destiny, sin, and astral influences played as great a part as any physical cause. The efficacy of cures was similarly bound in the beliefs of patient and doctor rather than empirical evidence, so that *remedia physicalia* (physical remedies) were often subordinate to spiritual intervention.

1.1.1 Influences

Hippocratic medicine

The Western medical tradition often traces roots directly to the early Greek civilization, much like the foundation of all of Western society. The Greeks certainly laid the foundation for Western medical practice but much more of Western medicine can be traced to the Middle East, Germanic, and Celtic cultures. The Greek medical foundation comes from a collection of writings known today as the Hippocratic Corpus.[2] Remnants of the Hippocratic Corpus survive in modern medicine in forms like the "Hippocratic Oath" as in to "Do No Harm.[3]"

The Hippocratic Corpus, popularly attributed to an ancient Greek practitioner known as Hippocrates, lays out the basic approach to health care. Greek philosophers viewed the human body as a system that reflects the workings nature and Hippocrates applied this belief to medicine. The body, as a reflection of natural forces, contained four elemental properties expressed to the Greeks as the four humors. The humors represented fire, air, earth and water through the properties of hot, cold, dry and moist, respectively.[4] Health in the human body relied on keeping these humors in balance within each person.

Maintaining the humors within a patient occurred in several ways. The primary tool of the physician to balance the patient's humors. An initial examination took place as standard for a physician to properly evaluate the patient. The patient's home climate, their normal diet, and astrological

1

charts were regarded during consultation. The heavens influenced every person in different ways by influencing elements connected to certain humors, important information in reaching a diagnosis. The physician could determine which humor was unbalanced in the patient and prescribe a new diet to restore that balance.[5] Diet not only included food to eat or avoid but also an exercise regiment and medication.

Hippocratic medicine represented learned medical practice beginning with the Hippocratic Corpus having been written down so practitioners had to be literate.[6] The written treatises within the Corpus are varied, incorporating medical doctrine from any source the Greeks came into contact with. At Alexandria in Egypt the Greeks learned the art of surgery and dissection, the Egyptian skill in these arenas far surpassed those of Greeks and Romans due to social taboos on the treatment of the dead.[7] The early Hippocratic practitioner Herophilus engaged in dissection and added new knowledge to human anatomy in the realms of the human nervous system, the inner workings of the eye, differentiating arteries from veins, and using pulses as a diagnostic tool in treatment.[8] Surgery and dissection yielded much knowledge of the human body that Hippocratic physicians employed alongside their methods of balancing humors in patients. The combination of knowledge in diet, surgery, and medication formed the foundation of medical learning upon which Galen would later greatly contribute.

Temple healing

The Greeks clearly had been influenced by their Egyptian neighbors in terms of medical practice in surgery and medication but the Greeks also absorbed many folk healing practices including incantations and dream healing. In Homer's Iliad and Odyssey the gods are implicated as the cause of plagues or widespread disease and that those maladies could be cured by praying to them. This religious side of healing clearly manifested in the cult of Asclepius, whom Homer regarded as the great physician, and was deified in the third and fourth century BC.[9] Hundreds of temples devoted to Asclepius have been found throughout the Greek and Roman empire to which untold numbers of people have flocked for cures. Healing visions and dreams formed the foundation for the curing process as the person seeking treatment from Asclepius slept in a special dormitory. The healing occurred either in the person's dream or advice from the dream could be used to seek out proper treatment for illness elsewhere. After wards the visitor to the temple bathed, offered prayers and sacrifice, and received other forms of treatment like medication, dietary restrictions, and an exercise regiment, keeping with the Hippocratic tradition.[10]

Pagan and folk medicine

Medicine in the Middle Ages had its roots in pagan and folk practices. This influence was highlighted by the interplay between Christian theologians who adopted aspects of pagan and folk practices and chronicled them in their own works. The practices adopted by Christian medical practitioners around the 2nd century, and their attitudes toward pagan and folk traditions, reflected an understanding of these practices, especially humoralism and herbalism. The practices of Christian medicine stemmed from pagan and folk practices.

The practice of medicine in the early Middle Ages was in fact empirical and pragmatic. It focused mainly on curing disease rather than discovering the cause of diseases.[11] Often it was believed the cause of disease was supernatural. Nevertheless, approaches to curing disease existed. People in the Middle Ages considered medicine through an understanding of the humors. This approach was likely influenced by a largely rural existence in which people understood the influences of the elements of the sustenance of agriculture. Since it was clear that the fertility of the earth depended on the proper balance of the elements, it followed that the same was true for the body, within which the various humors, as they were understood, had to be in balance.[12] This approach greatly influenced medical theory throughout the Middle Ages.

Folk medicine of the Middle Ages ostensibly dealt with the use of herbal remedies for ailments. The practice of keeping gardens teeming with various herbs with medicinal properties was a traditional practice influenced in medieval Europe by the gardens of Roman antiquity.[11] Many early medieval manuscripts have been noted for containing practical descriptions for the use of herbal remedies. These texts, such as the Pseudo-Apuleius, included illustrations various plants that would have been easily identifiable and familiar to Europeans at the time.[11] Monasteries later became centers of medical practice in the Middle Ages and carried on the tradition of maintaining gardens containing medicinal herbs. Herb gardens contained plants with healing properties. These gardens became specialized and capable of maintaining plants from Southern Hemispheres as well as maintaining plants during winter.[11] The practice of gardening for the purpose of supplying the ingredients necessary in medieval herbal medicinals was influenced by a rural folk tradition.

Again, that Europe in the early Middle Ages was largely rural and agricultural influenced folk medical practices at the time. Hildegard of Bingen was an example of a medieval medical practitioner who took her cues from this folk medical tradition. Her understanding of the elements in nature informed her commentary on the humors of the body and the remedies she described in her medical text,

Causae et curae, were greatly influenced by her familiarity with folk treatments of disease. In the rural society of Hildegard's time, much of the medical care was provided by women, along with their other domestic duties. Not surprisingly, their kitchen were stocked full of the herbs and other substances required in folk remedies for many ailments.[12] Causae et curae illustrated a view of symbiosis of the body and nature, that the understanding of nature could inform medical treatment of the body. However, Hildegard maintained the belief that the root of disease was a compromised relationship between a person and God.[12] Many parallels between pagan and Christian ideas about disease existed during the early Middle Ages. Many viewed medicine as being part of the natural order and therefore sought medical help for illness. Most of the focus of this early medicine remained focused on cures for rather than the causes of diseases. Christian views of disease differed from those held by pagans because of a fundamental difference in belief: Christians' belief in a personal relationship with God greatly influenced their views on medicine.[13] However, in spite of this key difference, Christian medical practitioners gave much credence to pagan tradition.

Evidence of pagan influence on emerging Christian medical practice was provided by many prominent early Christian thinkers, such as Origen, Clement, and Augustine, who studied natural philosophy and held important aspects of secular Greek philosophy that were in line with Christian thought. They believed faith supported by sound philosophy was superior to simple faith.[13] Other similarities between Christian and pagan views on medicine existed. Christian ideas about the role of physicians were influenced by previous pagan ideals. The classical idea of the physician as a selfless servant who had to endure unpleasant tasks and provide necessary, often painful treatment was of great influence on early Christian practitioners. The metaphor was not lost on Christians who viewed Christ as the ultimate physician.[13] Another similarity shared with the pagan perspective was the view of the relationship between disease and the individual. Pagan philosophy had previously held that the pursuit of virtue should not be secondary to bodily concerns. Similarly, Christians felt that, while caring for the body was important, it was second to spiritual pursuits.[13] Early Christianity was eager, for the most part, to borrow these certain aspects of pagan classical philosophy.

The practice of medicine in medieval Europe was longstanding. A classical pagan view of medicine in which the main focus was on treating and curing disease survived as the practice of medicine evolved through the Middle Ages. People in medieval Europe had long been practicing folk medicine as evidenced by the tradition of the herb garden. The continued practice of gardening in monasteries later on and the practicality and accessibility of the works of Hildegard of Bingen and other, as mentioned previously, illus-

trated a longstanding precedent of medical practice. The roots of medieval medicine in the pagan and folk medicine that preceded it illustrate a development of medical practice that took place in Europe over a long period of time.

Monasteries

Monasteries developed not only as spiritual centers, but also centers of intellectual learning and medical practice. Locations of the monasteries were secluded and designed to be self-sufficient, which required the monastic inhabitants to produce their own food and also care for their sick. Prior to the development of hospitals, people from the surrounding towns looked to the monasteries for help with their sick.

A combination of both spiritual and natural healing was used to treat the sick. Herbal remedies, known as Herbals, along with prayer and other religious rituals were used in treatment by the monks and nuns of the monasteries. Herbs were seen by the monks and nuns as one of God's creations for the natural aid that contributed to the spiritual healing of the sick individual. An herbal textual tradition also developed in the medieval monasteries.[14] Older herbal Latin texts were translated and also expanded in the monasteries. The monks and nuns, reorganized older texts so that the text could utilized more efficiently, adding a table of contents for example to help find information quickly. Not only did they reorganize existing texts, but they also added or eliminated information. New herbs that were discovered to be useful or specific herbs that were known in a particular geographic area were added. Herbs that proved to be ineffective were eliminated. Drawings were also added or modified in order for the reader to effectively identify the herb. The Herbals that were being translated and modified in the monasteries were some of the first medical texts produced and used in medical practice in the Middle Ages.[15]

Not only were herbal texts being produced, but also other medieval texts that discussed the importance and imbalance of the humors.Hildegard of Bingen, a well known abbess, wrote about Hippocratic Medicine using humoral theory and how balance and imbalance of the elements affected the health of an individual along with other known sicknesses of the time, and ways in which to combine both prayer and herbs form nature to help the individual become well. She discusses different symptoms that were common to see and the known remedies for them.[16]

In exchanging the herbal texts among monasteries, monks became aware of herbs that could be very useful but were not found in the surrounding area. The monastic clergy traded with one another or used commercial means to obtain the foreign herbs.[17] Inside most of the monastery grounds there had been a separate garden designated for the plants that were needed for the treatment of the sick.

A serving plan of St. Gall depicts a separate garden to be developed for strictly medical herbals.[18] Monks and nuns also devoted a large amount of their time in the cultivation of the herbs they felt were necessary in the care of the sick. Some plants were not native to the local area and needed special care to be kept alive. The monks used a form of science, what we would consider today, botany to cultivate these plants. Foreign herbs and also plants determined to be highly valuable were grown in gardens with in close proximity to the monastery in order for the monastic clergy to hastily have access to the natural remedies.

Medicine in the monasteries was concentrated on assisting the individual to return to normal health. Being able to identify symptoms and remedies was the primary focus. In some instances identifying the symptoms led the monastic clergy to have to take into consideration the cause of the illness in order to implement a solution. Research and experimental processes were continuously being implemented in monasteries to be able to successful fulfill their duties to God to take care of all God's people.

Christian charity

By AD 400 a community without a healer was, by Jewish law, no proper community. The Jews took their duty to care for their fellow Jews seriously. This duty extended to lodging and medical treatment of pilgrims to the temple at Jerusalem.[19] Temporary medical assistance had been provided in classical Greece for visitors to festivals and the tradition extended through the Roman empire, especially after Christianity became the state religion prior to its decline. In the early Medieval period hospitals, poor houses, hostels, and orphanages began to spread from the Middle East, each with the intention of helping those most in need.[20]

Charity, the driving principle behind these healing centers, encouraged the early Christians to care for others. The cities of Jerusalem, Constantinople, and Antioch contained some of the earliest and most complex hospitals with many beds to house patients and staff physicians with emerging specialties.[21] Some hospitals were large enough to provide education in medicine, surgery and patient care. St. Basil (AD 330-79) argued that God put medicines on the Earth for human use, while many early church fathers agreed that Hippocratic medicine could be used to treat the sick and satisfy the charitable need to help others.[22]

Medicine

Medieval European medicine became more developed during the Renaissance of the 12th century, when many medical texts both on Ancient Greek medicine and on Islamic medicine were translated from Arabic during the 13th century. The most influential among these texts was Avicenna's *The Canon of Medicine*, a medical encyclopedia written in *circa* 1030 which summarized the medicine of Greek, Indian and Muslim physicians until that time. The *Canon* became an authoritative text in European medical education until the early modern period. Other influential texts from Arabic authors include *De Gradibus* by Alkindus, the *Liber pantegni* by Isaac Israeli ben Solomon, and *Al-Tasrif'* *by Abulcasis*.

At Schola Medica Salernitana in Southern Italy, medical texts from Byzantium and the Arab world (see Medicine in medieval Islam) were readily available, translated from the Greek and Arabic at the nearby monastic centre of Monte Cassino. The Salernitan masters gradually established a canon of writings, known as the *ars medicinae* (art of medicine) or *articella* (little art), which became the basis of European medical education for several centuries.

During the Crusades the influence of Islamic medicine became stronger. The influence was mutual and Islamic scholars such as Usamah ibn Munqidh also described their experience with European medicine positive - he describes a European doctor successfully treating infected wounds with vinegar and recommends a treatment for scrofula demonstrated to him by an unnamed "Frank".[23]

Classical medicine

Anglo-Saxon translations of classical works like Dioscorides *Herbal* survive from the 10th century, showing the persistence of elements of classical medical knowledge. Other influential translated medical texts at the time included the Hippocratic Corpus attributed to Hippocrates, and the writings of Galen.

Galen of Pergamon, a Greek, was one of the most influential ancient physicians. Galen described the four classic symptoms of inflammation (redness, pain, heat, and swelling) and added much to the knowledge of infectious disease and pharmacology. His anatomic knowledge of humans was defective because it was based on dissection of animals, mainly apes, sheep, goats and pigs.[24] Some of Galen's teachings held back medical progress. His theory, for example, that the blood carried the pneuma, or life spirit, which gave it its red colour, coupled with the erroneous notion that the blood passed through a porous wall between the ventricles of the heart, delayed the understanding of circulation and did much to discourage research in physiology. His most important work, however, was in the field of the form and function of muscles and the function of the areas of the spinal cord. He also excelled in diagnosis and prognosis.

Medieval surgery

Early medieval surgery traces its roots to ancient times in Egyptian and Greek societies. One of the earliest influences on early European surgery was the great physician Galen. He was the first to incorporate the practice of dissection and many other types of surgical operations.

The emergence of universities in western Europe brought about the study of medicine as a focus of learning. The University of Padua and the University of Bologna were two Italian universities that focused on the study of medicine. The students from these schools would spend years working for a degree in medicine.

During the Crusades, surgeons would go around a battlefield to determine whether wounded soldiers were dead or alive. Some surgeons became specialized in removing arrowheads from their patients' bodies[25] Barber surgeons could be found in any medieval town and would mainly cut beards and hair. On occasion these men would be called for doing small operations like bloodletting (the practice of taking small quantities of blood to prevent illness or disease) or treating sword and arrow wounds. When doing operations on patients, doctors would only use anesthetics on patients who could pay for them. Most of the time patients would be given a piece of wood or leather to bite down on during the surgical procedure.

A special procedure known as trepanning (boring a hole in the skull) was used for patients who suffered from cerebral pressure or mental illnesses. Deep wounds that could not be closed otherwise were often seared closed by cauterization. Amputation was a procedure used to remove the limbs of a patient to stop future disease. Amputation was a violent practice that often caused problems for the patient later. During these procedures many patients would die either from shock due to blood loss or later infections of the operated area.

1.1.2 Important medieval contributions

Though it is not readily recognized the Middle Ages contributed a great deal to medical knowledge. This period contained progress in surgery, medical chemistry, dissection, and practical medicine. While there might not be a huge monumental event, the Middle Ages laid the ground work for later larger discoveries. There was a slow but constant progression in the way that medicine was studied and practiced. It went from apprenticeships to universities and from oral traditions to documenting texts. The most well-known preservers of texts, not only medical, would be the monasteries. The monks were able to copy and revise any medical texts that they were able to obtain. Besides documentation the Middle Ages also had one of the first well

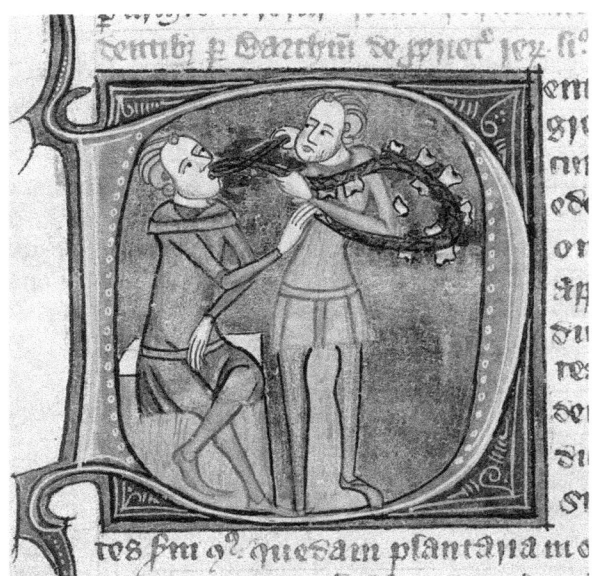

A dentist with silver forceps and a necklace of large teeth, extracting the tooth of a well seated man. Omne Bonum *(England - London; 1360–1375).*

known female physicians, Hildegard of Bingen.

Hildegard was born in 1098 and at the age of fourteen she entered the double monastery of Dissibodenberg.[26] She wrote the medical text Causae et curae in which many medical practices of the time were demonstrated. This book contained diagnosis, treatment, and prognosis of many different diseases and illnesses. This text was able to shed light on medieval medical practices of the time. It also shows the vast amount of knowledge and influences that she had available that she mentioned in her works. In this time period medicine was taken very seriously and it is shown with Hildegard's detailed descriptions on how to perform medical tasks.[27] The descriptions are nothing without their practical counterpart and Hildegard was thought to have been an infirmarian in the monastery where she lived. An infirmarian treated not only other monks but pilgrims, workers, and the poor men, women, and children in the monastery's hospice. Because monasteries were located in rural areas the infirmarian was also responsible for the care of lacerations, fractures, dislocations, and burns.[28] Along with typical medical practice the text also hints that the youth (such as Hildegard) would have received hands-on training from the previous infirmarian. Beyond routine nursing this also shows that medical remedies from plants, that were either grown or gathered, was something that had a significant impact of the future of medicine. This was the beginnings of the domestic pharmacy.[29]

Although plants were the main source of medieval remedies, around the sixteenth century medical chemistry became more prominent. "Medical chemistry began with the adaptation of chemical processes to the preparation of medicine".[30] Previously medical chemistry was characterized by any use of inorganic materials, but it was later refined to be more technical, like the processes of distillation. John of Rupescissa's works in alchemy and the beginnings of medical chemistry is recognized for the bounds in chemistry. His works in making the philosopher's stone, also known as the fifth essence, was what made him well known.[31] Distillation techniques were mostly used and it was said that by reaching a substance's purest form the person would find the fifth essence, and this is where medicine comes in. Remedies were able to be made more potently because there was now a way to remove nonessential extras. This opened many doors for medieval physicians because new, different remedies were being made. Medical chemistry provided an "increasing body of pharmacological literature dealing with the use of medicines derived from mineral sources".[32] Medical chemistry also shows the use alcohols in medicine and though these events were not huge bounds it was influential in determining the course of science. It was the start of differentiation between alchemy and chemistry.

The Middle Ages brought a new way of thinking and a lessening on the taboo of dissection. Dissection for medical purposes became more prominent around 1299.[33] During this time the Italians were practicing anatomical dissection and the first record of an autopsy dates from 1286. Dissection was first introduced in the educational setting at the university of Bologna to study and teach anatomy. The fourteenth century was the huge spread of dissection and autopsy in Italy and was not only taken up by medical faculties, but by colleges for physicians and surgeons.[34]

The founding of the Universities of Paris (1150), Bologna (1158), Oxford, (1167), Montpelier (1181) and Padua (1222), extended the initial work of Salerno across Europe, and by the thirteenth century medical leadership had passed to these newer institutions. To qualify as a Doctor of Medicine took ten years including original Arts training, and so the numbers of such fully qualified physicians remained comparatively small.

Roger Frugardi of Parma composed his treatise on *Surgery* around about 1180. Between 1350 and 1365 Theodoric Borgognoni produced a systematic four volume treatise on surgery, the *Cyrurgia*, which promoted important innovations as well as early forms of antiseptic practice in the treatment of injury, and surgical anaesthesia using a mixture of opiates and herbs.

Compendiums like Bald's *Leechbook* (circa 900), include citations from a variety of classical works alongside local folk remedies.

1.1.3 Theories of medicine

Although each of these theories has distinct roots in different cultural and religious traditions, they were all intertwined in the general understanding and practice of medicine. For example, the Benedictine abbess and healer, Hildegard of Bingen, claimed that black bile and other humour imbalances were directly caused by presence of the devil and by sin.[35] Another example of the fusion of different medicinal theories is the combination of Christian and pre-Christian ideas about *elf-shot* (elf- or fairy-caused diseases) and their appropriate treatments. The idea that elves caused disease was a pre-Christian belief that developed into the Christian idea of disease-causing demons or devils.[36] Treatments for this and other types of illness reflected the coexistence of Christian and pre-Christian or pagan ideas of medicine.

Humours

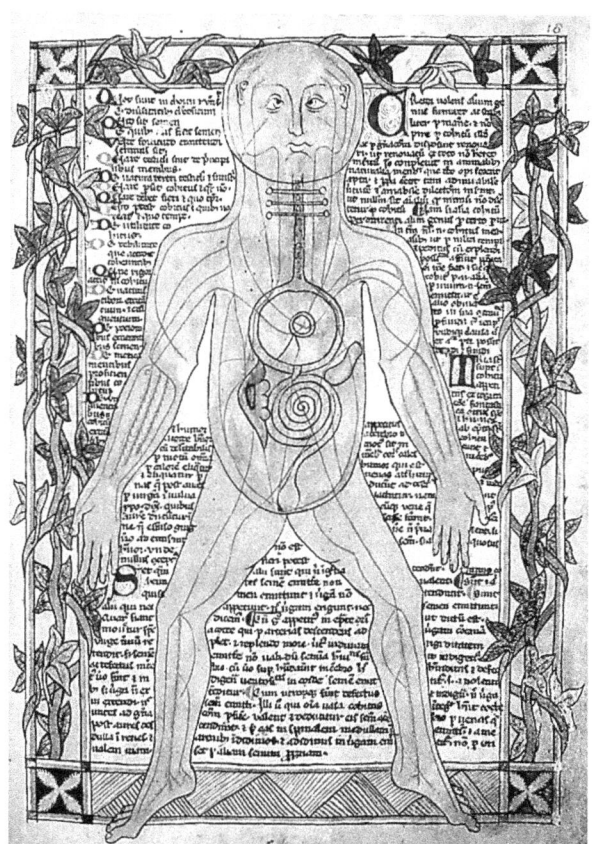

13th-century illustration showing the veins.

Main article: Humorism

The underlying principle of medieval medicine was the theory of humours. This was derived from the ancient medical works, and dominated all western medicine until the 19th century. The theory stated that within every individual there were four **humours**, or principal fluids - black bile, yellow bile, phlegm, and blood, these were produced by various organs in the body, and they had to be in balance for a person to remain healthy. Too much phlegm in the body, for example, caused lung problems; and the body tried to cough up the phlegm to restore a balance. The balance of humours in humans could be achieved by diet, medicines, and by blood-letting, using leeches. The four humours were also associated with the four seasons, black bile-autumn, yellow bile-summer, phlegm-winter and blood-spring.

The astrological signs of the zodiac were also thought to be associated with certain humours. Even now, some still use words "choleric", "sanguine", "phlegmatic" and "melancholy" to describe personalities.

Herbalism

Main article: Herbalism

Herbs were commonly used in salves and drinks to treat a range of maladies. The particular herbs used depended largely on the local culture and often had roots in pre-Christian religion.[36] The success of herbal remedies was often ascribed to their action upon the humours within the body. The use of herbs also drew upon the medieval Christian doctrine of signatures which stated that God had provided some form of alleviation for every ill, and that these things, be they animal, vegetable or mineral, carried a mark or a *signature* upon them that gave an indication of their usefulness. For example, skullcap seeds (used as a headache remedy) can appear to look like miniature skulls; and the white spotted leaves of lungwort (used for tuberculosis) bear a similarity to the lungs of a diseased patient. A large number of such resemblances were believed to exist.

Many monasteries developed herb gardens for use in the production of herbal cures,[37] and these remained a part of folk medicine, as well as being used by some professional physicians. Books of herbal remedies were produced, one of the most famous being the Welsh, *Red Book of Hergest*, dating from around 1400.

Christian interpretation of illness and continued influence

Medicine in the Middle Ages was rooted in Christianity through not only the spread of medical texts through monastic tradition but also through the beliefs of sickness in conjunction with medical treatment and theory. The church taught that God sometimes sent illness as a punishment,

and that in these cases, repentance could lead to a recovery. This led to the practice of penance and pilgrimage as a means of curing illness. In the Middle Ages, some people did not consider medicine a profession suitable for Christians, as disease was often considered God-sent. God was considered to be the "divine physician" who sent illness or healing depending on his will. From a Christian perspective disease could be seen either as a punishment from God or as an affliction of demons (or elves, see first paragraph under Theories of Medicine). The ultimate healer in this interpretation is of course God, but medical practitioners cited both the bible and Christian history as evidence that humans could and should attempt to cure diseases. For example, the Lorsch Book of Remedies or the Lorsch Leechbook contains a lengthy defense of medical practice from a Christian perspective. Christian treatments focused on the power of prayer and holy words, as well as liturgical practice.[38]

However, many monastic orders, particularly the Benedictines, were very involved in healing and caring for the sick and dying.[39] In many cases, the Greek philosophy that early Medieval medicine was based upon was compatible with Christianity.[40] Though the widespread Christian tradition of sickness being a divine intervention in reaction to sin was popularly believed throughout the Middle Ages, it did not rule out natural causes. For example, the Black Death was thought to have been caused by both divine and natural origins.[41] The plague was thought to have been a punishment from God for sinning, however because it was believed that God was the reason for all natural phenomena, the physical cause of the plague could be scientifically explained as well. One of the more widely accepted scientific explanations of the plague was the corruption of air in which pollutants such as rotting matter or anything that gave the air an unpleasant scent caused the spread of the plague.[42]

Hildegard of Bingen played an important role in how illness was interpreted through both God and natural causes through her medical texts as well. As a nun, she believed in the power of God and prayer to heal, however she also recognized that there were natural forms of healing through the humors as well. Though there were cures for illness outside of prayer, ultimately the patient was in the hands of God.[43] One specific example of this comes from her text *Causae et Curae* in which she explains the practice of bleeding:

> Bleeding, says Hildegard, should be done when the moon is waning, because then the "blood is low" (77:23-25). Men should be bled from the age of twelve (120:32) to eighty (121:9), but women, because they have more of the detrimental humors, up to the age of one hundred (121:24). For therapeutic bleeding, use the veins

nearest the diseased part (122:19); for preventive bleeding, use the large veins in the arms (121:35-122:11), because they are like great rivers whose tributaries irrigate the body (123:6-9, 17-20). 24 From a strong man, take "the amount that a thirsty person can swallow in one gulp" (119:20); from a weak one, "the amount that an egg of moderate size can hold" (119:22-23). Afterward, let the patient rest for three days and give him undiluted wine (125:30), because "wine is the blood of the earth" (141:26). This blood can be used for prognosis; for instance, "if the blood comes out turbid like a man's breath, and if there are black spots in it, and if there is a waxy layer around it, then the patient will die, unless God restore him to life" (124:20-24).[43]

Monasteries were also important in the development of hospitals throughout the Middle Ages, where the care of sick members of the community was an important obligation. These monastic hospitals weren't only for the monks who lived at the monasteries but also the pilgrims, visitors and surrounding population.[41] The monastic tradition of herbals and botany influenced Medieval medicine as well, not only in their actual medicinal uses but in their textual traditions. Texts on herbal medicine were often copied in monasteries by monks but there is substantial evidence that these monks were also practicing the texts that they were copying. These texts were progressively modified from one copy to the next, with notes and drawings added into the margins as the monks learned new things and experimented with the remedies and plants that the books supplied.[44] Monastic translations of texts continued to influence medicine as many Greek medical works were translated into Arabic. Once these Arabic texts were available, monasteries in western Europe were able to translate them, which in turn would help shape and redirect western medicine in the later Middle Ages.[45] The ability for these texts to spread from one monastery or school in adjoining regions created a rapid diffusion of medical texts throughout western Europe.[46]

The influence of Christianity continued on into the later periods of the Middle Ages as medical training and practice moved out of the monasteries and into cathedral schools, though more for the purpose of general knowledge rather than training professional physicians. The study of medicine was eventually institutionalized into the medieval universities.[41] Even within the university setting, religion dictated a lot of the medical practice being taught.For instance, the debate of when the spirit left the body influenced the practice of dissection within the university setting. The universities in the South believed that the soul only animated the body and left immediately upon death. Because of this, the body while still important, went from being a

subject to an object. However, in the north they believed that it took longer for the soul to leave as it was an integral part of the body.[47] Though medical practice had become a professional and institutionalized field, the argument of the soul in the case of dissection shows that the foundation of religion was still an important part of medical thought in the late Middle Ages.

1.1.4 Medical practitioners

Members of religious orders were major sources of medical knowledge and cures. There appears to have been some controversy regarding the appropriateness of medical practice for members of religious orders. The Decree of the Second Lateran Council of 1139 advised the religious to avoid medicine because it was a well-paying job with higher social status than was appropriate for the clergy. However, this official policy was not often enforced in practice and many religious continued to practice medicine.[37]

There were many other medical practitioners besides clergy. Academically trained doctors were particularly important in cities with universities. Medical faculty at universities figured prominently in defining medical guilds and accepted practices as well as the required qualifications for physicians.[37] Beneath these university-educated physicians there existed a whole hierarchy of practitioners. Wallis suggests a social hierarchy with these university educated physicians on top, followed by "learned surgeons; craft-trained surgeons; barber surgeons, who combined bloodletting with the removal of "superfluities" from the skin and head; itinernant specialist such as dentist and oculists; empirics; midwives; clergy who dispensed charitable advice and help; and, finally, ordinary family and neighbors".[37] Each of these groups practiced medicine in their own capacity and contributed to the overall culture of medicine.

1.1.5 Hospital system

In the Medieval period the term *hospital* encompassed hostels for travellers, dispensaries for poor relief, clinics and surgeries for the injured, and homes for the blind, lame, elderly, and mentally ill. Monastic hospitals developed many treatments, both therapeutic and spiritual.

During the thirteenth century an immense number of hospitals were built. The Italian cities were the leaders of the movement. Milan had no fewer than a dozen hospitals and Florence before the end of the fourteenth century had some thirty hospitals. Some of these were very beautiful buildings. At Milan a portion of the general hospital was designed by Bramante and another part of it by Michelangelo. The Hospital of Sienna, built in honor of St. Catherine, has been famous ever since. Everywhere throughout Europe this hospital movement spread. Virchow, the great German pathologist, in an article on hospitals, showed that every city of Germany of five thousand inhabitants had its hospital. He traced all of this hospital movement to Pope Innocent III, and though he was least papistically inclined, Virchow did not hesitate to give extremely high praise to this pontiff for all that he had accomplished for the benefit of children and suffering mankind.[48]

Hospitals began to appear in great numbers in France and England. Following the French Norman invasion into England, the explosion of French ideals led most Medieval monasteries to develop a hospitium or hospice for pilgrims. This hospitium eventually developed into what we now understand as a hospital, with various monks and lay helpers providing the medical care for sick pilgrims and victims of the numerous plagues and chronic diseases that afflicted Medieval Western Europe. Benjamin Gordon supports the theory that the hospital – as we know it - is a French invention, but that it was originally developed for isolating lepers and plague victims, and only later undergoing modification to serve the pilgrim.[49]

Owing to a well-preserved 12th-century account of the monk Eadmer of the Canterbury cathedral, there is an excellent account of Bishop Lanfranc's aim to establish and maintain examples of these early hospitals:

> But I must not conclude my work by omitting what he did for the poor outside the walls of the city Canterbury. In brief, he constructed a decent and ample house of stone...for different needs and conveniences. He divided the main building into two, appointing one part for men oppressed by various kinds of infirmities and the other for women in a bad state of health. He also made arrangements for their clothing and daily food, appointing ministers and guardians to take all measures so that nothing should be lacking for them.[50]

1.1.6 Later developments

High medieval surgeons like Mondino de Liuzzi pioneered anatomy in European universities and conducted systematic human dissections. Unlike pagan Rome, high medieval Europe did not have a complete ban on human dissection. However, Galenic influence was still so prevalent

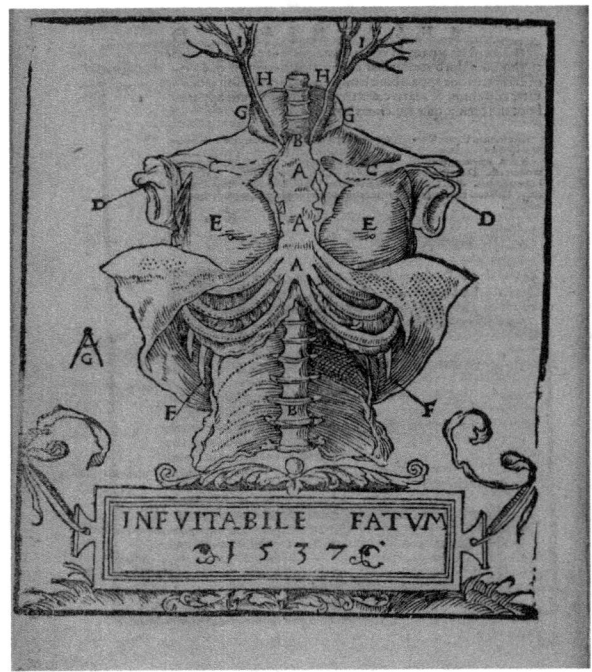

Anathomia, *1541*

that Mondino and his contemporaries attempted to fit their human findings into Galenic anatomy.

During the period of the Renaissance from the mid 1450s onward, there were many advances in medical practice. The Italian Girolamo Fracastoro(1478–1553) was the first to propose that epidemic diseases might be caused by objects outside the body that could be transmitted by direct or indirect contact.[51] He also proposed new treatments for diseases such as syphilis.

In 1543 the Flemish Scholar Andreas Vesalius wrote the first complete textbook on human anatomy: "De Humani Corporis Fabrica", meaning "On the Fabric of the Human Body". Much later, in 1628, William Harvey explained the circulation of blood through the body in veins and arteries. It was previously thought that blood was the product of food and was absorbed by muscle tissue.

During the 16th century, Paracelsus, like Girolamo, discovered that illness was caused by agents outside the body such as bacteria, not by imbalances within the body.

The French army doctor Ambroise Paré, born in 1510, revived the ancient Greek method of tying off blood vessels. After amputation the common procedure was to cauterize the open end of the amputated appendage to stop the haemorrhaging. This was done by heating oil, water, or metal and touching it to the wound to seal off the blood vessels. Pare also believed in dressing wounds with clean bandages and ointments, including one he made himself composed

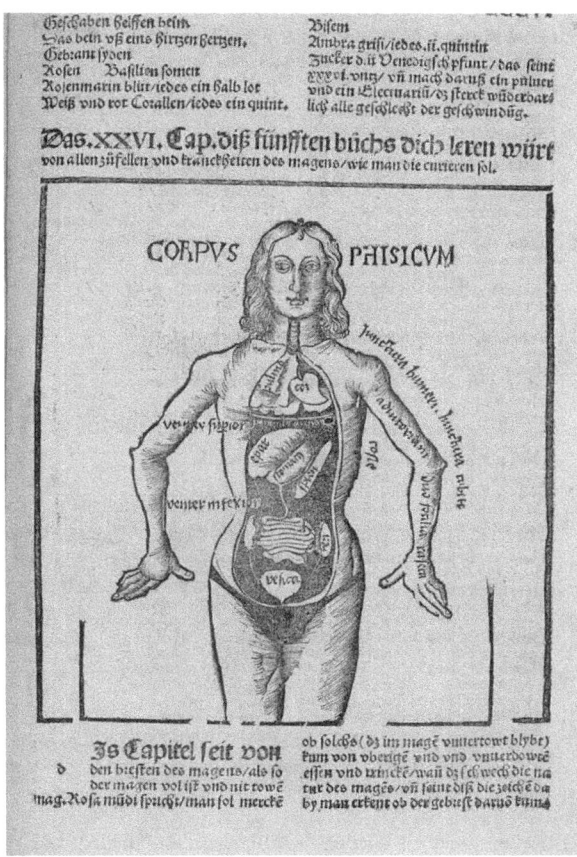

Corpus physicum, from Liber de arte Distillandi de Compositis, *1512*

of eggs, oil of roses, and turpentine. He was the first to design artificial hands and limbs for amputation patients. On one of the artificial hands, the two pairs of fingers could be moved for simple grabbing and releasing tasks and the hand look perfectly natural underneath a glove.

Medical catastrophes were more common in the late Middle Ages and the Renaissance than they are today. During the Renaissance, trade routes were the perfect means of transportation for disease. Eight hundred years after the Plague of Justinian, the bubonic plague returned to Europe. Starting in Asia, the Black Death reached Mediterranean and western Europe in 1348 (possibly from Italian merchants fleeing fighting in Crimea), and killed 25 million Europeans in six years, approximately 1/3 of the total population and up to a 2/3 in the worst-affected urban areas. Before Mongols left besieged Crimean Kaffa the dead or dying bodies of the infected soldiers were loaded onto catapults and launched over Kaffa's walls to infect those inside. This incident was among the earliest known examples of biological warfare and is credited as being the source of the spread of the Black Death into Europe.

The plague repeatedly returned to haunt Europe and the Mediterranean from 14th through 17th centuries. Notable later outbreaks include the Italian Plague of 1629–1631, the Great Plague of Seville (1647–1652), the Great Plague of London (1665–1666), the Great Plague of Vienna (1679), the Great Plague of Marseille in 1720–1722 and the 1771 plague in Moscow.

Before the Spanish discovered the new world (continental America), the deadly infections of smallpox, measles, and influenza were unheard of. The Native Americans did not have the immunities the Europeans developed through long contact with the diseases. Christopher Columbus ended the Americas' isolation in 1492 while sailing under the flag of Castile, Spain. Deadly epidemics swept across the Caribbean. Smallpox wiped out villages in a matter of months. The island of Hispaniola had a population of 250,000 Native Americans. 20 years later, the population had dramatically dropped to 6,000. 50 years later, it was estimated that approximately 500 Native Americans were left. Smallpox then spread to the area which is now Mexico where it then helped destroy the Aztec Empire. In the 1st century of Spanish rule in what is now Mexico, 1500–1600, Central and South Americans died by the millions. By 1650, the majority of New Spain (now Mexico) population had perished.

Contrary to popular belief[52] bathing and sanitation were not lost in Europe with the collapse of the Roman Empire.[53][54] Bathing in fact did not fall out of fashion in Europe until shortly after the Renaissance, replaced by the heavy use of sweat-bathing and perfume, as it was thought in Europe that water could carry disease into the body through the skin. Medieval church authorities believed that public bathing created an environment open to immorality and disease. Roman Catholic Church officials even banned public bathing in an unsuccessful effort to halt syphilis epidemics from sweeping Europe.[55]

1.1.7 See also

- Beak doctor costume
- Byzantine medicine
- History of hospitals
- History of medicine
- History of nursing
- Ibn Sina Academy of Medieval Medicine and Sciences
- Irish medical families
- Islamic medicine
- Life expectancy

- Medieval demography

- Plague doctor

- Plague doctor contract

- Theriac

1.1.8 Footnotes

[1] *Anthropologie structurale*, Lévi-Strauss, Claude (1958, Structural Anthropology, trans. Claire Jacobson and Brooke Grundfest Schoepf, 1963)

[2] Lawrence Conrad, Michael Neve, Vivian Nutton, Roy Porter, Andrew Wear. The Western Medical Tradition 800 BC to AD 1800. Cambridge University Press, New York, 1995, p16–17

[3] Nutton, The Western Medical Tradition, p19

[4] Nutton, The Western Medical Tradition, p25

[5] Nutton, The Western Medical Tradition, p23-25

[6] Lindberg, David C. The Beginnings of Western Science: The European Scientific Tradition in Philosophical, Religious, and Institutional Context, Prehistory to A.D. 1450. University of Chicago Press, Chicago and London, 2007, p118

[7] Lindberg, The Beginnings of Western Science, p119

[8] Lindberg, The Beginnings of Western Science, p120

[9] Lindberg, The Beginnings of Western Science, p111

[10] Lindberg, The Beginnings of Western Science, p112-113

[11] Voigts, Linda (June 1, 1979). "Anglo-Saxon Plant Remedies and the Anglo-Saxons". *Isis* **70** (2): 250–268. doi:10.1086/352199.

[12] Sweet, Victoria (1999). "Hildegard of Bingen and the Greening of Medieval Medicine". *Bulletin of the History of Medicine* **73** (3): 381–403. doi:10.1353/bhm.1999.0140. PMID 10500336.

[13] Amundsen, Darrel, W. (1982). "Medicine and Faith in Early Christianity". *Bulletin of the History of Medicine* **56** (3): 326–350. PMID 6753984.

[14] Voigts, Linda. "Anglo-Saxon Plant Remedies and the Anglo-Saxons. The University of Chicago Press, 1979. p. 251

[15] Voigts, Linda. "Anglo-Saxon Plant Remedies and the Anglo-Saxons. The University of Chicago Press, 1979. p. 253

[16] Sweet, Victoria. "Hildegard of Binger and the Greening of Medieval Medicine". The Johns Hopkins University Press, 1999

[17] Voigts, Linda. "Anglo-Saxon Plant Remedies and the Anglo-Saxons. The University of Chicago Press, 1979. p. 259

[18] Voigts, Linda. "Anglo-Saxon Plant Remedies and the Anglo-Saxons. The University of Chicago Press, 1979. p. 265

[19] Nutton, The Western Medical Tradition, p73-74

[20] Nutton, The Western Medical Tradition, p79

[21] Nutton, The Western Medical Tradition, p78

[22] St. Basil the Great on the Art of Medicine

[23] Medieval Sourcebook: Usmah Ibn Munqidh (1095–1188): *Autobiography*, excerpts on the Franks.

[24] Nutton, Vivian; Lawrence I. Conrad; Michael Neve; Roy Porter; Andrew Wear (1995). *The Western Medical Tradition: 800 B.C.–1800 A.D.* Cambridge: Cambridge University Press. p. 66. ISBN 0-521-38135-5.

[25] Bellerby, Rachel. "Surgery in Medieval Times". Retrieved 2014-05-12.

[26] Sweet, Victoria (1999). "Hildegard of Bingen and the Greening of Medieval Medicine". *Bulletin of the History of Medicine* **73** (3): 381–403. doi:10.1353/bhm.1999.0140. PMID 10500336.

[27] Sweet, Victoria (1999). "Hildegard of Bingen and the Greening of Medieval Medicine". *Bulletin of the History of Medicine* **73** (3): 389. doi:10.1353/bhm.1999.0140.

[28] Sweet, Victoria (1999). "Hildegard of Bingen and the Greening of Medieval Medicine". *Bulletin of the History of Medicine* **73** (3): 396. doi:10.1353/bhm.1999.0140.

[29] Sweet, Victoria (1999). "Hildegard of Bingen and the Greening of Medieval Medicine". *Bulletin of the History of Medicine* **73** (3): 399. doi:10.1353/bhm.1999.0140.

[30] Multhauf, Robert (1954). "John of Rupescissa and the Origin of Medical Chemistry". *Isis* **45** (4): 359. doi:10.1086/348357.

[31] Multhauf, Robert (1954). "John of Rupescissa and the Origin of Medical Chemistry". *Isis* **45** (4): 360. doi:10.1086/348357.

[32] Multhauf, Robert (1954). "John of Rupescissa and the Origin of Medical Chemistry". *Isis* **45** (4): 366. doi:10.1086/348357.

[33] Park, Katharine (1995). "The Life of the Corpse: Division and Dissection in Late Medieval Europe". *Journal of the History of Medicine and Allied Sciences* **50**: 113. doi:10.1093/jhmas/50.1.111.

[34] Park, Katharine (1995). "The Life of the Corpse: Division and Dissection in Late Medieval Europe". *Journal of the History of Medicine and Allied Sciences* **50**: 114. doi:10.1093/jhmas/50.1.111.

[35] *Causes and Cures*. Berlin: Akademie Verlag. 2003. |first1= missing |last1= in Authors list (help)

[36] Jolly, Karen Louise (1996). *Popular Religion in Late Saxon England: Elf Charms in Context*. Chapel Hill: The University of North Carolina Press.

[37] Wallis, Faith (2010). *Medieval Medicine: A Reader*. Toronto: University of Toronto Press.

[38] Jolly, Karen Louise (1996). *Popular Religion in Late Saxon England: Elf Charms in Context*. Chapel Hill: The University of North Carolina Press.

[39] Wallis, Faith (2010). Medieval Medicine: A Reader. Toronto: University of Toronto Press.

[40] Amundsen, Darrel W. (1982). "Medicine and Faith in Early Christianity". *Bulletin of the History of Medicine* **56** (3): 326–50.

[41] Lindberg, D. C. (2007). Medieval Medicine and Natural History. The beginnings of western science: the European scientific tradition in philosophical, religious, and institutional context, prehistory to A.D. 1450 (2nd ed.,). Chicago: University of Chicago Press.

[42] Horrox, R. (1994). The Black Death. Manchester: Manchester University Press.

[43] Sweet, V. (1999). "Hildegard of bingen and the greening of medieval medicine". *Bulletin of the history of Medicine* **73** (3): 381–403. doi:10.1353/bhm.1999.0140. PMID 10500336.

[44] Voigts L. E. (1979). "Anglo-Saxon Plant Remedies and the Anglo-Saxons". *Isis* **70** (2): 250–268. doi:10.1086/352199. JSTOR 230791.

[45] Lindberg, D. C. (2007). Medieval Medicine and Natural History. The beginnings of western science: the European scientific tradition in philosophical, religious, and institutional context, prehistory to A.D. 1450 (2nd ed.,). Chicago: University of Chicago Press. p 327

[46] Lindberg, D. C., & Talbot, C. H. (1978). Medicine. Science in the Middle Ages (). Chicago: University of Chicago Press. p. 403.

[47] Park, K. (1995). The Life of the Corpse: Division and Dissection in Late Medieval Europe. Journal of the History of Medicine and Allied Sciences, 50, 111–132.

[48] Walsh, James Joseph (1924). *The world's debt to the Catholic Church*. The Stratford Company. p. 244.

[49] Gordon, Benjamin (1959). *Medieval and Renaissance Medicine*. New York: Philosophical Library. p. 341.

[50] Orme, Nicholas (1995). *The English Hospital: 1070–1570*. New Haven: Yale Univ. Press. pp. 21–22.

[51] Fracastoro, Girolamo. *De Contagione*.

[52] The Bad Old Days — Weddings & Hygiene

[53] The Great Famine (1315–1317) and the Black Death (1346–1351)

[54] Middle Ages Hygiene

[55] Paige, John C; Laura Woulliere Harrison (1987). *Out of the Vapors: A Social and Architectural History of Bathhouse Row, Hot Springs National Park* (PDF). U.S. Department of the Interior.

1.1.9 Further reading

- Bowers, Barbara S. ed. *The Medieval Hospital and Medical Practice* (Ashgate, 2007); 258pp; essays by scholars

- Getz, Faye. *Medicine in the English Middle Ages.* (Princeton University Press, 1998). ISBN 0-691-08522-6

- Mitchell, Piers D. *Medicine in the Crusades: Warfare, Wounds, and the Medieval Surgeon* (Cambridge University Press, 2004) 293 pp.

- Porter, Roy. *The Greatest Benefit to Mankind. A medical history of humanity from antiquity to the present.* (HarperCollins 1997)

- Siraisi Nancy G (2012). "Medicine, 1450–1620, and the History of Science". *Isis* **103** (3): 491–514. doi:10.1086/667970. PMID 23286188.

Primary sources

- Wallis, Faith, ed. *Medieval Medicine: A Reader* (2010) excerpt and text search

1.1.10 External links

- Medieval Medicine

- "Index of Medieval Medical Images" UCLA Special Collections (accessed 2 September 2006).

- "The Wise Woman" An overview of common ailments and their treatments from the Middle Ages presented in a slightly humorous light.

- "MacKinney Collection of Medieval Medical Illustrations"

- PODCAST: Professor Peregrine Horden (Royal Holloway University of London): 'What's wrong with medieval medicine?'

- Walsh, James J. *Medieval Medicine*(1920), A & C Black, Ltd.

- Interactive game with medieval diseases and cures

- Encyclopedic manuscript containing allegorical and medical drawings From the Rare Book and Special Collections Division at the Library of Congress

Chapter 2

History of Medieval Medicine

2.1 Black Death

For other uses, see Black Death (disambiguation).

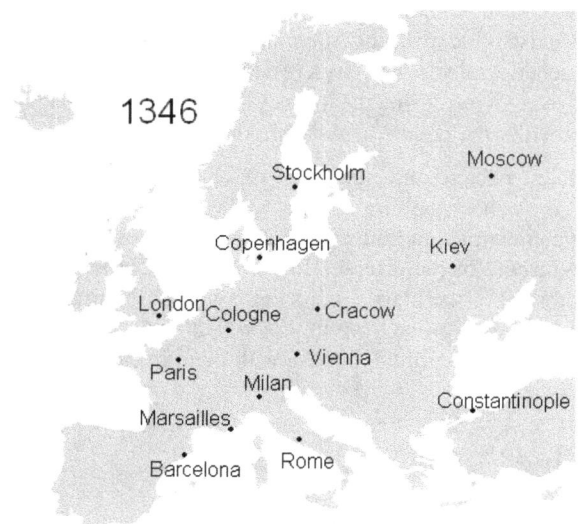

1346

Spread of the Black Death in Europe (1346–53)

The **Black Death** was one of the most devastating pandemics in human history, resulting in the deaths of an estimated 75 to 200 million people and peaking in Europe in the years 1346–53.[1][2][3] Although there were several competing theories as to the etiology of the Black Death, analysis of DNA from victims in northern and southern Europe published in 2010 and 2011 indicates that the pathogen responsible was the *Yersinia pestis* bacterium, probably causing several forms of plague.[4][5]

The Black Death is thought to have originated in the arid plains of Central Asia, where it then travelled along the Silk Road, reaching Crimea by 1343.[6] From there, it was most likely carried by Oriental rat fleas living on the black rats that were regular passengers on merchant ships. Spreading throughout the Mediterranean and Europe, the Black Death is estimated to have killed 30–60% of Europe's total population.[7] In total, the plague reduced the world population from an estimated 450 million down to 350–375 million in the 14th century. The world population as a whole did not recover to pre-plague levels until the 17th century.[8] The plague recurred occasionally in Europe until the 19th century.

The plague created a series of religious, social, and economic upheavals, which had profound effects on the course of European history.

2.1.1 Chronology

Origins of the disease

Main article: Black Death migration

The plague disease, caused by *Yersinia pestis*, is enzootic (commonly present) in populations of fleas carried by ground rodents, including marmots, in various areas including Central Asia, Kurdistan, Western Asia, Northern India and Uganda.[9] Nestorian graves dating to 1338–9 near Lake Issyk Kul in Kyrgyzstan have inscriptions referring to plague and are thought by many epidemiologists to mark the outbreak of the epidemic, from which it could easily have spread to China and India.[10] In October 2010, medical geneticists suggested that all three of the great waves of the plague originated in China.[11] In China, the 13th century Mongol conquest caused a decline in farming and trading. However, economic recovery had been observed at the beginning of the 14th century. In the 1330s a large number of natural disasters and plagues led to widespread famine, starting in 1331, with a deadly plague arriving soon after.[12] Epidemics which may have included plague killed an estimated 25 million Chinese and other Asians during the 15 years before it reached Constantinople in 1347.[13][14]

The disease may have travelled along the Silk Road with Mongol armies and traders or it could have come via ship.[15] By the end of 1346, reports of plague had reached the seaports of Europe: "India was depopulated, Tartary, Mesopotamia, Syria, Armenia were covered with dead bodies".[16]

Plague was reportedly first introduced to Europe via Genoese traders at the port city of Kaffa in the Crimea in 1347. After a protracted siege, during which the Mongol army under Jani Beg was suffering from the disease, the army catapulted the infected corpses over the city walls of Kaffa to infect the inhabitants. The Genoese traders fled, taking the plague by ship into Sicily and the south of Europe, whence it spread north.[17] Whether or not this hypothesis is accurate, it is clear that several existing conditions such as war, famine, and weather contributed to the severity of the Black Death.

European outbreak

The seventh year after it began, it came to England and first began in the towns and ports joining on the seacoasts, in Dorsetshire, where, as in other counties, it made the country quite void of inhabitants so that there were almost none left alive.
... But at length it came to Gloucester, yea even to Oxford and to London, and finally it spread over all England and so wasted the people that scarce the tenth person of any sort was left alive.

Geoffrey the Baker, *Chronicon Angliae*

There appear to have been several introductions into Europe. The plague reached Sicily in October 1347, carried by twelve Genoese galleys,[18] and rapidly spread all over the island. Galleys from Kaffa reached Genoa and Venice in January 1348, but it was the outbreak in Pisa a few weeks later that was the entry point to northern Italy. Towards the end of January, one of the galleys expelled from Italy arrived in Marseille.[19]

From Italy, the disease spread northwest across Europe, striking France, Spain, Portugal and England by June 1348, then turned and spread east through Germany and Scandinavia from 1348 to 1350. It was introduced in Norway in 1349 when a ship landed at Askøy, then spread to Bjørgvin (modern Bergen) and Iceland.[20] Finally it spread to northwestern Russia in 1351. The plague was somewhat less common in parts of Europe that had smaller trade relations with their neighbours, including the Kingdom of Poland, the majority of the Basque Country, isolated parts of Belgium and the Netherlands, and isolated alpine villages throughout the continent.[21][22]

Modern researchers do not think that the plague ever became endemic in Europe or its rat population. The disease repeatedly wiped out the rodent carriers so that the fleas died out until a new outbreak from Central Asia repeated the process. The outbreaks have been shown to occur roughly 15 years after a warmer and wetter period in areas where plague is endemic in other species such as gerbils.[23][24]

Middle Eastern outbreak

The plague struck various countries in the Middle East during the pandemic, leading to serious depopulation and permanent change in both economic and social structures. As it spread to western Europe, the disease entered the region from southern Russia also. By autumn 1347, the plague reached Alexandria in Egypt, probably through the port's trade with Constantinople, and ports on the Black Sea. During 1347, the disease travelled eastward to Gaza, and north along the eastern coast to cities in Lebanon, Syria and Palestine, including Ashkelon, Acre, Jerusalem, Sidon, Damascus, Homs, and Aleppo. In 1348–49, the disease reached Antioch. The city's residents fled to the north, most of them dying during the journey, but the infection had been spread to the people of Asia Minor.

Mecca became infected in 1349. During the same year, records show the city of Mawsil (Mosul) suffered a massive epidemic, and the city of Baghdad experienced a second round of the disease. In 1351 Yemen experienced an outbreak of the plague, coinciding with the return of King Mujahid of Yemen from imprisonment in Cairo. His party may have brought the disease with them from Egypt.

2.1.2 Symptoms

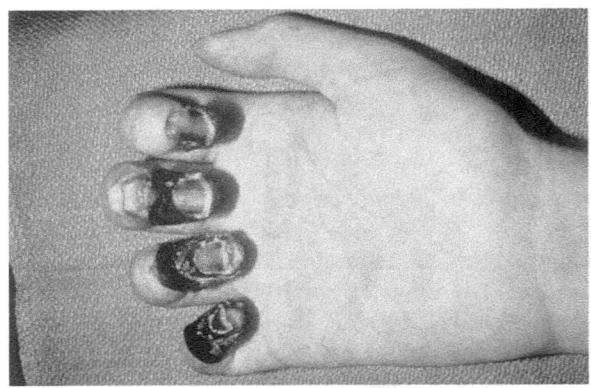

A hand showing how acral gangrene of the fingers due to bubonic plague causes the skin and flesh to die and turn black

Contemporary accounts of the plague are often varied or imprecise. The most commonly noted symptom was the appearance of buboes (or gavocciolos) in the groin, the neck

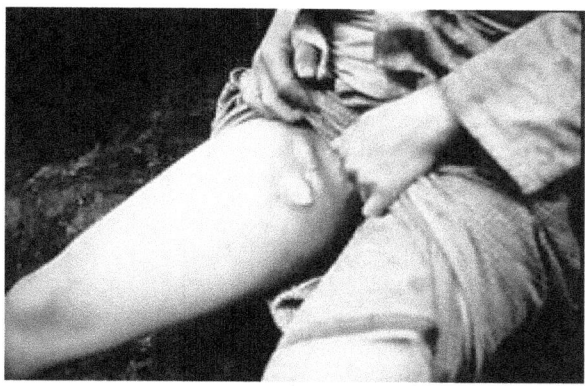

An inguinal bubo on the upper thigh of a person infected with bubonic plague. Swollen lymph glands (buboes) often occur in the neck, armpit and groin (inguinal) regions of plague victims

and armpits, which oozed pus and bled when opened.[25] Boccaccio's description is graphic:

> In men and women alike it first betrayed itself by the emergence of certain tumours in the groin or armpits, some of which grew as large as a common apple, others as an egg...From the two said parts of the body this deadly gavocciolo soon began to propagate and spread itself in all directions indifferently; after which the form of the malady began to change, black spots or livid making their appearance in many cases on the arm or the thigh or elsewhere, now few and large, now minute and numerous. As the gavocciolo had been and still was an infallible token of approaching death, such also were these spots on whomsoever they showed themselves.[26]

The only medical detail that is questionable is the infallibility of approaching death, as if the bubo discharges, recovery is possible.[27]

This was followed by acute fever and vomiting of blood. Most victims died two to seven days after initial infection. Freckle-like spots and rashes[28] which could be caused by flea-bites as another potential sign of the plague.

Some accounts, like that of Louis Heyligen, a musician in Avignon who died of the plague in 1348, noted a distinct form of the disease which infected the lungs and led to respiratory problems[25] and which is identified with pneumonic plague.

> It is said that the plague takes three forms. In the first people suffer an infection of the lungs, which leads to breathing difficulties. Whoever

has this corruption or contamination to any extent cannot escape but will die within two days. Another form...in which boils erupt under the armpits,...a third form in which people of both sexes are attacked in the groin.[29]

2.1.3 Naming

The phrase "black death" (*atra mors*) is ancient, derived from Homeric Greek[30] and adopted in classical Latin. It is in origin a poetic characterisation of death as dark and terrible (*ater* "black" having the overtones of "gloomy, sad, dismal, unlucky") not used specifically of epidemics or the bubonic plague. The 12th-century French physician Gilles de Corbeil in his *De signis et sinthomatibus egritudinum* (On the signs and symptoms of diseases) used it to refer to a pestilential fever (*febris pestilentialis*) [31]

Writers contemporary to the plague referred to the event as the "Great Mortality",[32] or the "Great Plague".[33] The phrase "Black Death" (*mors nigra*) is used in 1350 by Simon de Covino (or Couvin), a Belgian astronomer, who wrote the poem "*De judicio Solis in convivio Saturni*" (On the judgment of the Sun at a feast of Saturn) in which he attributed the plague to a conjunction of Jupiter and Saturn.[34]

Gasquet (1908) claimed that the Latin name *atra mors* (Black Death) for the 14th-century epidemic first appeared in modern times in 1631 in a book on Danish history by J.I. Pontanus: "*Vulgo & ab effectu* atram mortem *vocatibant.* ("Commonly and from its effects, they called it the black death").[35] The name spread through Scandinavia and then Germany, gradually becoming attached to the mid 14th-century epidemic as a proper name.[36] In England, it was not until 1823 that the medieval epidemic was first called the Black Death.[37]

2.1.4 Causes

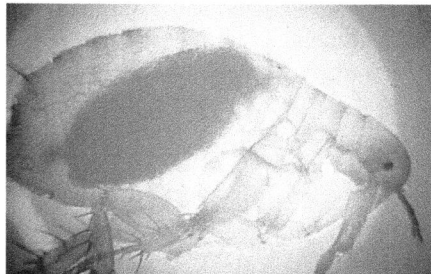

The Oriental rat flea (*Xenopsylla cheopis*) engorged with blood after a blood meal. This species of flea is the primary vector for the transmission of *Yersinia pestis*, the organism responsible for bubonic plague in most plague epidemics.

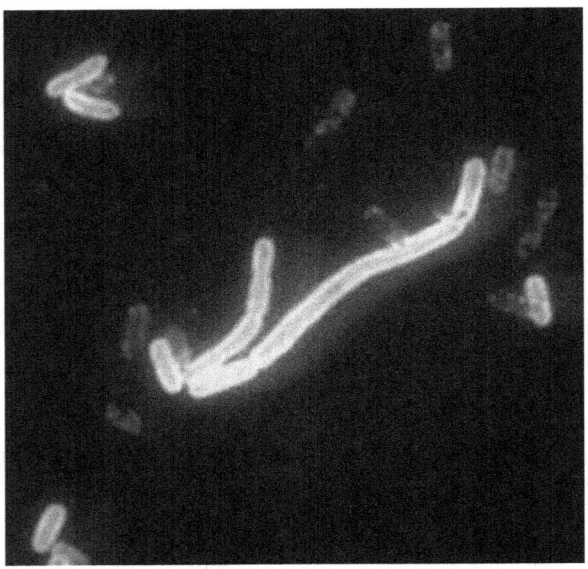

Yersinia pestis *(200x magnification). The bacterium which causes bubonic plague.*[38]

Both male and female fleas feed on blood and can transmit the infection.

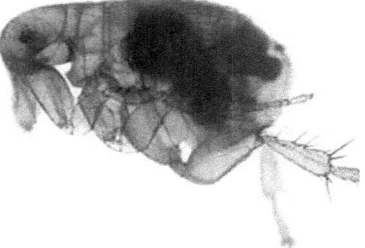

Oriental rat flea (*Xenopsylla cheopis*) infected with the *Yersinia pestis* bacterium which appears as a dark mass in the gut. The foregut (*proventriculus*) of this flea is blocked by a *Y. pestis* biofilm; when the flea attempts to feed on an uninfected host *Y. pestis* is regurgitated into the wound, causing infection.

Medical knowledge had stagnated during the Middle Ages. The most authoritative account at the time came from the medical faculty in Paris in a report to the king of France that blamed the heavens, in the form of a conjunction of three planets in 1345 that caused a "great pestilence in the air".[39] This report became the first and most widely circulated of a series of plague tracts that sought to give advice to sufferers. That the plague was caused by bad air became the most widely accepted theory. The word 'plague' had no special significance at this time, and only the recurrence of outbreaks during the Middle Ages gave it the name that has become the medical term.

The importance of hygiene was recognised only in the nine-

teenth century; until then it was common that the streets were filthy, with live animals of all sorts around and human parasites abounding. A transmissible disease will spread easily in such conditions. One development as a result of the Black Death was the establishment of the idea of quarantine in Dubrovnik in 1377 after continuing outbreaks.[40]

The dominant explanation for the Black Death is the plague theory, which attributes the outbreak to *Yersinia pestis*, also responsible for an epidemic that began in southern China in 1865, eventually spreading to India. The investigation of the pathogen that caused the 19th-century plague was begun by teams of scientists who visited Hong Kong in 1894, among whom was the French-Swiss bacteriologist Alexandre Yersin, after whom the pathogen was named *Yersinia pestis*.[41] The mechanism by which *Y. pestis* was usually transmitted was established in 1898 by Paul-Louis Simond and was found to involve the bites of fleas whose midguts had become obstructed by replicating *Y. pestis* several days after feeding on an infected host. This blockage results in starvation and aggressive feeding behaviour by the fleas, which repeatedly attempt to clear their blockage by regurgitation, resulting in thousands of plague bacteria being flushed into the feeding site, infecting the host. The bubonic plague mechanism was also dependent on two populations of rodents: one resistant to the disease, which act as hosts, keeping the disease endemic, and a second that lack resistance. When the second population dies, the fleas move on to other hosts, including people, thus creating a human epidemic.[41]

The historian Francis Aidan Gasquet, who had written about the 'Great Pestilence' in 1893[42] and suggested that "it would appear to be some form of the ordinary Eastern or bubonic plague" was able to adopt the epidemiology of the bubonic plague for the Black Death for the second edition in 1908, implicating rats and fleas in the process, and his interpretation was widely accepted for other ancient and medieval epidemics, such as the Justinian plague that was prevalent in the Eastern Roman Empire from 541 to 700 CE.[41]

Other forms of plague have been implicated by modern scientists. The modern bubonic plague has a mortality rate of 30–75% and symptoms including fever of 38–41 °C (100–106 °F), headaches, painful aching joints, nausea and vomiting, and a general feeling of malaise. Left untreated, of those that contract the bubonic plague, 80 percent die within eight days.[43] Pneumonic plague has a mortality rate of 90 to 95 percent. Symptoms include fever, cough, and blood-tinged sputum. As the disease progresses, sputum becomes free flowing and bright red. Septicemic plague is the least common of the three forms, with a mortality rate near 100%. Symptoms are high fevers and purple skin patches (purpura due to disseminated intravascular coagulation). In cases of pneumonic and particularly septicemic plague the progress of the disease is so rapid that there would often be no time for the development of the enlarged lymph nodes that were noted as buboes.[44]

DNA evidence

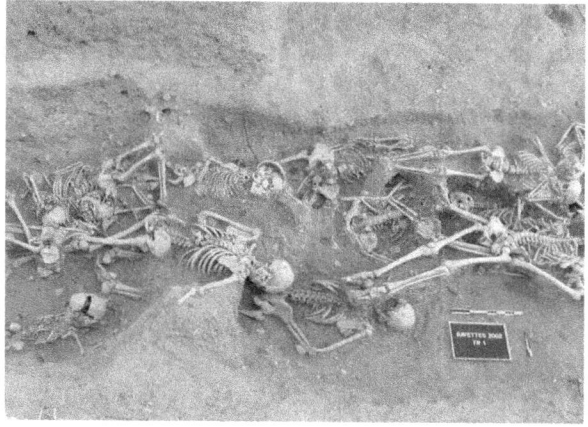

Skeletons in a mass grave from 1720–1721 in Martigues, France, yielded molecular evidence of the orientalis *strain of* Yersinia pestis, *the organism responsible for bubonic plague. The second pandemic of bubonic plague was active in Europe from AD 1347, the beginning of the Black Death, until 1750.*

In October 2010, the open-access scientific journal *PLoS Pathogens* published a paper by a multinational team who undertook a new investigation into the role of *Yersinia pestis* in the Black Death following the disputed identification by Drancourt and Raoult in 1998.[45] Their surveys tested for DNA and protein signatures specific for *Y. pestis* in human skeletons from widely distributed mass graves in northern, central and southern Europe that were associated archaeologically with the Black Death and subsequent resurgences. The authors concluded that this new research, together with prior analyses from the south of France and Germany

> ...ends the debate about the etiology of the Black Death, and unambiguously demonstrates that *Y. pestis* was the causative agent of the epidemic plague that devastated Europe during the Middle Ages.[46]

The study also found that there were two previously unknown but related clades (genetic branches) of the *Y. pestis* genome associated with medieval mass graves. These clades (which are thought to be extinct) were found to be ancestral to modern isolates of the modern *Y. pestis* strains *Y. p. orientalis* and *Y. p. medievalis*, suggesting the plague may have entered Europe in two waves. Surveys of plague pit remains in France and England indicate the first variant entered Europe through the port of Marseille around Novem-

ber 1347 and spread through France over the next two years, eventually reaching England in the spring of 1349, where it spread through the country in three epidemics. Surveys of plague pit remains from the Dutch town of Bergen op Zoom showed the *Y. pestis* genotype responsible for the pandemic that spread through the Low Countries from 1350 differed from that found in Britain and France, implying Bergen op Zoom (and possibly other parts of the southern Netherlands) was not directly infected from England or France in 1349 and suggesting a second wave of plague, different from those in Britain and France, may have been carried to the Low Countries from Norway, the Hanseatic cities or another site.[46]

The results of the Haensch study have since been confirmed and amended. Based on genetic evidence derived from Black Death victims in the East Smithfield burial site in England, Schuenemann et al. concluded in 2011 "that the Black Death in medieval Europe was caused by a variant of *Y. pestis* that may no longer exist."[47] A study published in *Nature* in October 2011 sequenced the genome of *Y. pestis* from plague victims and indicated that the strain that caused the Black Death is ancestral to most modern strains of the disease.[5]

DNA taken from 25 skeletons from the 14th century found in London have shown the plague is a strain of *Y. pestis* that is almost identical to that which hit Madagascar in 2013.[48][49]

Alternative explanations

Main article: Theories of the Black Death

The plague theory was first significantly challenged by the work of British bacteriologist J. F. D. Shrewsbury in 1970, who noted that the reported rates of mortality in rural areas during the 14th-century pandemic were inconsistent with the modern bubonic plague, leading him to conclude that contemporary accounts were exaggerations.[41] In 1984 zoologist Graham Twigg produced the first major work to challenge the bubonic plague theory directly, and his doubts about the identity of the Black Death have been taken up by a number of authors, including Samuel K. Cohn, Jr. (2002), David Herlihy (1997), and Susan Scott and Christopher Duncan (2001).[41]

It is recognised that an epidemiological account of the plague is as important as an identification of symptoms, but researchers are hampered by the lack of reliable statistics from this period. Most work has been done on the spread of the plague in England, and even estimates of overall population at the start vary by over 100% as no census was undertaken between the time of publication of the Domesday Book and the year 1377.[50] Estimates of plague victims are usually extrapolated from figures from the clergy.

In addition to arguing that the rat population was insufficient to account for a bubonic plague pandemic, sceptics of the bubonic plague theory point out that the symptoms of the Black Death are not unique (and arguably in some accounts may differ from bubonic plague); that transference via fleas in goods was likely to be of marginal significance and that the DNA results may be flawed and might not have been repeated elsewhere, despite extensive samples from other mass graves.[41] Other arguments include the lack of accounts of the death of rats before outbreaks of plague between the 14th and 17th centuries; temperatures that are too cold in northern Europe for the survival of fleas; that, despite primitive transport systems, the spread of the Black Death was much faster than that of modern bubonic plague; that mortality rates of the Black Death appear to be very high; that, while modern bubonic plague is largely endemic as a rural disease, the Black Death indiscriminately struck urban and rural areas; and that the pattern of the Black Death, with major outbreaks in the same areas separated by 5 to 15 years, differs from modern bubonic plague—which often becomes endemic for decades with annual flare-ups.[41]

Walløe complains that all of these authors "take it for granted that Simond's infection model, black rat → rat flea → human, which was developed to explain the spread of plague in India, is the only way an epidemic of *Yersinia pestis* infection could spread", whilst pointing to several other possibilities.[51]

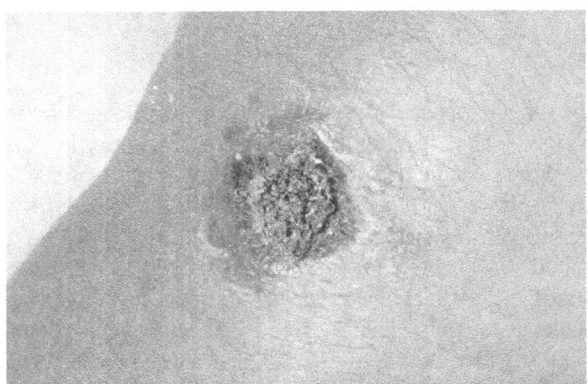

Anthrax skin lesion

A variety of alternatives to the *Y. pestis* have been put forward. Twigg suggested that the cause was a form of anthrax and N. F. Cantor (2001) thought it may have been a combination of anthrax and other pandemics. Scott and Duncan have argued that the pandemic was a form of infectious disease that characterise as *hemorrhagic* plague similar to Ebola. Archaeologist Barney Sloane has argued that there is insufficient evidence of the extinction of large number

of rats in the archaeological record of the medieval waterfront in London and that the plague spread too quickly to support the thesis that the *Y. pestis* was spread from fleas on rats and argues that transmission must have been person to person.[52][53] However, no single alternative solution has achieved widespread acceptance.[41] Many scholars arguing for the *Y. pestis* as the major agent of the pandemic suggest that its extent and symptoms can be explained by a combination of bubonic plague with other diseases, including typhus, smallpox and respiratory infections. In addition to the bubonic infection, others point to additional septicemic (a type of "blood poisoning") and pneumonic (an airborne plague that attacks the lungs before the rest of the body) forms of the plague, which lengthen the duration of outbreaks throughout the seasons and help account for its high mortality rate and additional recorded symptoms.[25] In 2014, scientists with Public Health England announced the results of an examination of 25 bodies exhumed from the Clerkenwell area of London, as well as of wills registered in London during the period, which supported the pneumonic hypothesis.[48]

2.1.5 Consequences

Main article: Consequences of the Black Death

Death toll

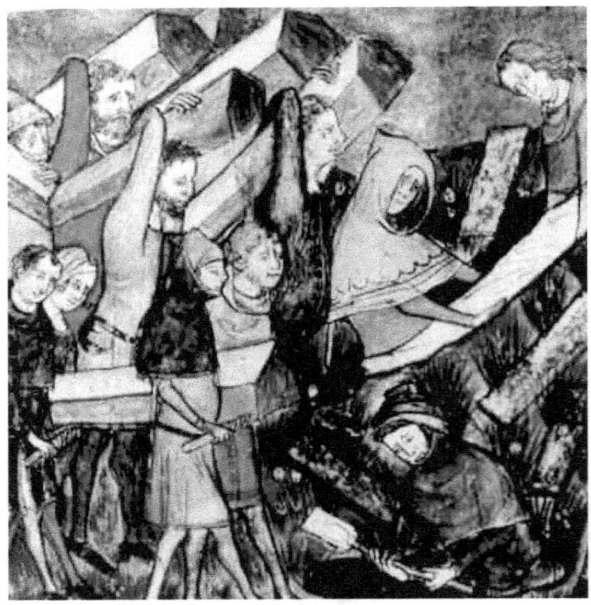

Citizens of Tournai bury plague victims.

There are no exact figures for the death toll; the rate varied widely by locality. It killed some 75 to 200 million people in Eurasia.[1][2][3] According to medieval historian Philip Daileader in 2007:

> The trend of recent research is pointing to a figure more like 45–50% of the European population dying during a four-year period. There is a fair amount of geographic variation. In Mediterranean Europe, areas such as Italy, the south of France and Spain, where plague ran for about four years consecutively, it was probably closer to 75–80% of the population. In Germany and England ... it was probably closer to 20%.[54]

The most widely accepted estimate for the Middle East, including Iraq, Iran and Syria, during this time, is for a death rate of about a third.[55] The Black Death killed about 40% of Egypt's population.[56] Half of Paris's population of 100,000 people died. In Italy, Florence's population was reduced from 110–120 thousand inhabitants in 1338 down to 50 thousand in 1351. At least 60% of Hamburg's and Bremen's population perished,[57] and a similar percentage of Londoners may have died from the disease as well.[48] Interestingly while contemporary reports account of mass burial pits being created in response to the large numbers of dead, recent scientific investigations of a burial pit in Central London found well-preserved individuals to be buried in isolated, evenly spaced graves, suggesting at least some pre-planning and Christian burials at this time.[58] Before 1350, there were about 170,000 settlements in Germany, and this was reduced by nearly 40,000 by 1450.[59] In 1348, the plague spread so rapidly that before any physicians or government authorities had time to reflect upon its origins, about a third of the European population had already perished. In crowded cities, it was not uncommon for as much as 50% of the population to die. The disease bypassed some areas, and the most isolated areas were less vulnerable to contagion. Monks and priests were especially hard hit since they cared for the Black Death's victims.[60]

Persecutions

See also: Black Death Jewish persecutions
Renewed religious fervor and fanaticism bloomed in the wake of the Black Death. Some Europeans targeted "various groups such as Jews, friars, foreigners, beggars, pilgrims",[61] lepers[61][62] and Romani, thinking that they were to blame for the crisis. Lepers, and other individuals with skin diseases such as acne or psoriasis, were singled out and exterminated throughout Europe.

Because 14th-century healers were at a loss to explain the cause, Europeans turned to astrological forces, earthquakes, and the poisoning of wells by Jews as possible reasons for

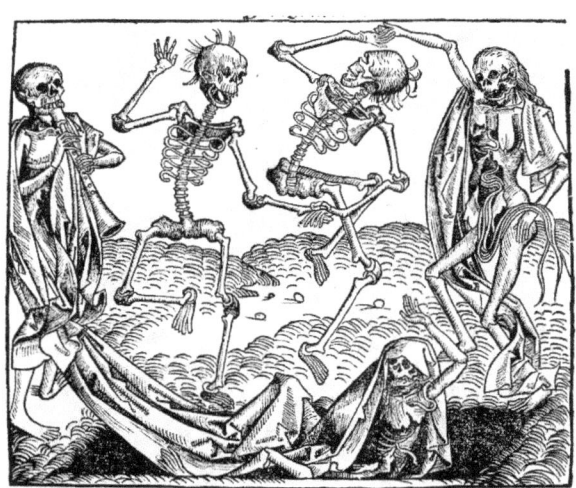

Inspired by the Black Death, The Dance of Death *or* Danse Macabre, *an allegory on the universality of death, is a common painting motif in the late medieval period.*

the plague's emergence.[33] The governments of Europe had no apparent response to the crisis because no one knew its cause or how it spread. The mechanism of infection and transmission of diseases was little understood in the 14th century; many people believed only God's anger could produce such horrific displays.

There were many attacks against Jewish communities.[63] In August 1349, the Jewish communities of Mainz and Cologne were exterminated. In February of that same year, the citizens of Strasbourg murdered 2,000 Jews.[63] By 1351, 60 major and 150 smaller Jewish communities were destroyed.[64]

Recurrence

Main article: Second plague pandemic
The plague repeatedly returned to haunt Europe and the Mediterranean throughout the 14th to 17th centuries.[65] According to Biraben, the plague was present somewhere in Europe in every year between 1346 and 1671.[66] The Second Pandemic was particularly widespread in the following years: 1360–63; 1374; 1400; 1438–39; 1456–57; 1464–66; 1481–85; 1500–03; 1518–31; 1544–48; 1563–66; 1573–88; 1596–99; 1602–11; 1623–40; 1644–54; and 1664–67. Subsequent outbreaks, though severe, marked the retreat from most of Europe (18th century) and northern Africa (19th century).[67] According to Geoffrey Parker, "France alone lost almost a million people to the plague in the epidemic of 1628–31."[68]

In England, in the absence of census figures, historians propose a range of preincident population figures from as high as 7 million to as low as 4 million in 1300,[69] and a postin-

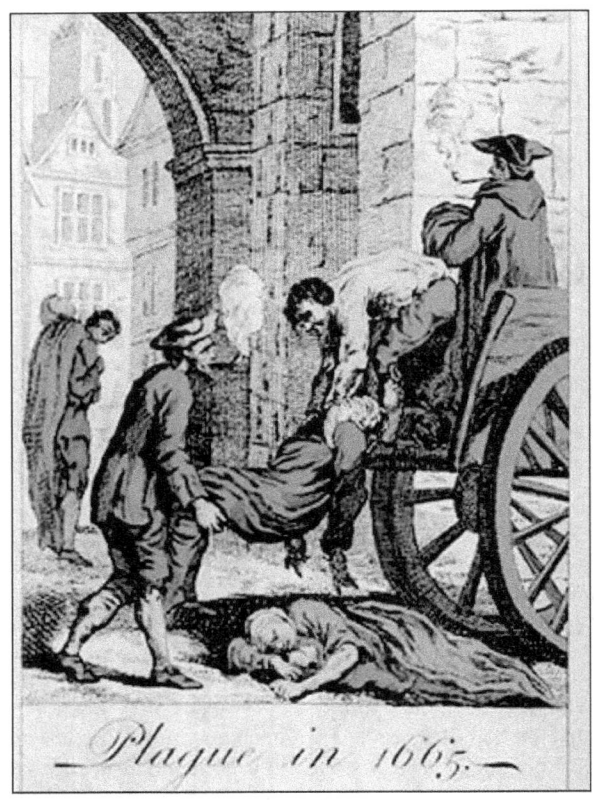

The Great Plague of London, in 1665, killed up to 100,000 people

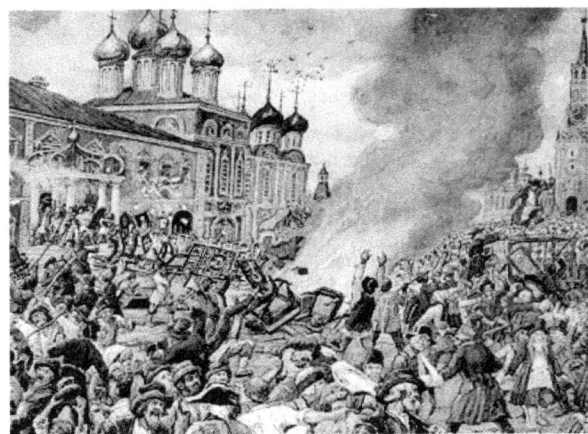

Plague Riot in Moscow in 1771: During the course of the city's plague, between 50 and 100 thousand people died, $\frac{1}{6}$ to $\frac{1}{3}$ of its population.

cident population figure as low as 2 million.[70] By the end of 1350, the Black Death subsided, but it never really died out in England. Over the next few hundred years, further outbreaks occurred in 1361–62, 1369, 1379–83, 1389–93, and throughout the first half of the 15th century.[71] An outbreak in 1471 took as much as 10–15% of the population, while the death rate of the plague of 1479–80 could have been as high as 20%.[72] The most general outbreaks in Tudor and Stuart England seem to have begun in 1498, 1535, 1543, 1563, 1589, 1603, 1625, and 1636, and ended with the Great Plague of London in 1665.[73]

In 1466, perhaps 40,000 people died of the plague in Paris.[74] During the 16th and 17th centuries, the plague was present in Paris around 30 per cent of the time.[75] The Black Death ravaged Europe for three years before it continued on into Russia, where the disease was present somewhere in the country 25 times between 1350 to 1490.[76] Plague epidemics ravaged London in 1563, 1593, 1603, 1625, 1636, and 1665,[77] reducing its population by 10 to 30% during those years.[78] Over 10% of Amsterdam's population died in 1623–25, and again in 1635–36, 1655, and 1664.[79] Plague occurred in Venice 22 times between 1361 and 1528.[80] The plague of 1576–77 killed 50,000 in Venice, almost a third of the population.[81] Late outbreaks in central Europe included the Italian Plague of 1629–1631,

which is associated with troop movements during the Thirty Years' War, and the Great Plague of Vienna in 1679. Over 60% of Norway's population died in 1348–50.[82] The last plague outbreak ravaged Oslo in 1654.[83]

In the first half of the 17th century, a plague claimed some 1.7 million victims in Italy, or about 14% of the population.[84] In 1656, the plague killed about half of Naples' 300,000 inhabitants.[85] More than 1.25 million deaths resulted from the extreme incidence of plague in 17th-century Spain.[86] The plague of 1649 probably reduced the population of Seville by half.[87] In 1709–13, a plague epidemic that followed the Great Northern War (1700–21, Sweden v. Russia and allies)[88] killed about 100,000 in Sweden,[89] and 300,000 in Prussia.[87] The plague killed two-thirds of the inhabitants of Helsinki,[90] and claimed a third of Stockholm's population.[91] Europe's last major epidemic occurred in 1720 in Marseille.[82]

World Distribution of Plague, 1998

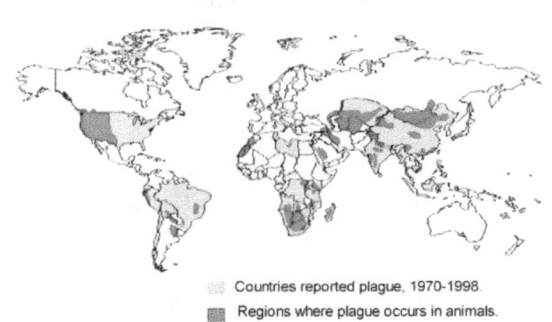

☐ Countries reported plague, 1970-1998.
▨ Regions where plague occurs in animals.

Worldwide distribution of plague-infected animals 1998

The Black Death ravaged much of the Islamic world.[92]

Plague was present in at least one location in the Islamic world virtually every year between 1500 and 1850.[93] Plague repeatedly struck the cities of North Africa. Algiers lost 30 to 50 thousand inhabitants to it in 1620–21, and again in 1654–57, 1665, 1691, and 1740–42.[94] Plague remained a major event in Ottoman society until the second quarter of the 19th century. Between 1701 and 1750, thirty-seven larger and smaller epidemics were recorded in Constantinople, and an additional thirty-one between 1751 and 1800.[95] Baghdad has suffered severely from visitations of the plague, and sometimes two-thirds of its population has been wiped out.[96]

Third plague pandemic

Main article: Third plague pandemic

The Third plague pandemic (1855–1859) started in China in the middle of the 19th century, spreading to all inhabited continents and killing 10 million people in India alone.[97] Twelve plague outbreaks in Australia in 1900–25 resulted in well over 1,000 deaths, chiefly in Sydney. This led to the establishment of a Public Health Department there which undertook some leading-edge research on plague transmission from rat fleas to humans via the bacillus *Yersinia pestis*.[98]

The first North American plague epidemic was the San Francisco plague of 1900–04, followed by another outbreak in 1907–08.[99] From 1944 through 1993, 362 cases of human plague were reported in the United States; approximately 90% occurred in four western states: Arizona, California, Colorado, and New Mexico.[100] Plague was confirmed in the United States from 9 western states during 1995.[101] Currently, 5 to 15 people in the United States are estimated to catch the disease each year—typically in western states.[102][103]

2.1.6   Treatment

Modern treatment methods include insecticides, the use of antibiotics, and a plague vaccine. The plague bacterium could develop drug-resistance and again become a major health threat. One case of a drug-resistant form of the bacterium was found in Madagascar in 1995.[104] A further outbreak in Madagascar was reported in November 2014.[105]

2.1.7   See also

- Black Death (film)

- Black Death in England

- CCR5, a human gene hypothesised to be associated with the plague

- *Cronaca fiorentina* (*Chronicle of Florence*); a literary history of the plague, and of Florence up to 1386, by Baldassarre Bonaiuti

- Crisis of the Late Middle Ages

- Danse Macabre

- Death

- Four thieves vinegar; a popular French legend says this recipe provided immunity to the plague.

- Geisslerlieder

- Globalization and disease

- Plague doctor

- Plague doctor costume

- Ring a Ring o' Roses

- *The Seventh Seal*, a film directed by Ingmar Bergman

2.1.8   References

[1] ABC/Reuters (29 January 2008). "Black death 'discriminated' between victims (ABC News in Science)". Australian Broadcasting Corporation. Retrieved 3 November 2008.

[2] "Health. De-coding the Black Death". BBC. 3 October 2001. Retrieved 3 November 2008.

[3] "Black Death's Gene Code Cracked". *Wired*. 3 October 2001. Retrieved 12 February 2015.

[4] Haensch S, Bianucci R, Signoli M, Rajerison M, Schultz M, Kacki S, Vermunt M, Weston DA, Hurst D, Achtman M, Carniel E, Bramanti B (2010). Besansky, Nora J, ed. "Distinct clones of Yersinia pestis caused the black death". *PLoS Pathog.* **6** (10): e1001134. doi:10.1371/journal.ppat.1001134. PMC 2951374. PMID 20949072.

[5] Bos KI, Schuenemann VJ, Golding GB, Burbano HA, Waglechner N, Coombes BK, McPhee JB, DeWitte SN, Meyer M, Schmedes S, Wood J, Earn DJ, Herring DA, Bauer P, Poinar HN, Krause J (12 October 2011). "A draft genome of Yersinia pestis from victims of the Black Death". *Nature* **478** (7370): 506–10. doi:10.1038/nature10549. PMC 3690193. PMID 21993626.

[6] "BBC – History – Black Death". BBC. 17 February 2011.

[7] Austin Alchon, Suzanne (2003). *A pest in the land: new world epidemics in a global perspective*. University of New Mexico Press. p. 21. ISBN 0-8263-2871-7.

[8] Wheeler, Dr. L. Kip. "The Black Plague: The Least You Need to Know". *Dr. Wheeler's website.* Dr. L. Kip Wheeler. Retrieved 9 August 2015.

[9] Ziegler 1998, p. 25.

[10] Raoult; Drancourt (2008). "Paleomicrobiology: Past Human Infections". Springer. p. 152.

[11] Nicholas Wade (31 October 2010). "Europe's Plagues Came From China, Study Finds". *The New York Times.* Retrieved 1 November 2010.

[12] The Cambridge History of China: Alien regimes and border states, 907–1368, p.585

[13] Kohn, George C. (2008). *Encyclopedia of plague and pestilence: from ancient times to the present.* Infobase Publishing. p. 31. ISBN 0-8160-6935-2.

[14] Sussman GD (2011). "Was the black death in India and China?". *Bulletin of the history of medicine* **85** (3): 319–55. doi:10.1353/bhm.2011.0054. PMID 22080795.

[15] "Black Death may have originated in China". *The Daily Telegraph.* 1 November 2010.

[16] Hecker 1859, p. 21 cited by Ziegler, p. 15.

[17] "Channel 4 – History – The Black Death". Channel 4. Archived from the original on 25 June 2008. Retrieved 3 November 2008.

[18] Michael of Piazza (Platiensis) *Bibliotheca scriptorum qui res in Sicilia gestas retulere* Vol 1, p. 562, cited in Ziegler, 1998, p. 40.

[19] De Smet, Vol II, *Breve Chronicon*, p. 15.

[20] Gunnar Karlsson (2000). *Iceland's 1100 years: the history of a marginal society.* London:C. Hurst. p. 111. ISBN 978-1-85065-420-9.

[21] Zuchora-Walske, Christine, Poland, North Mankato: ABDO Publishing, 2013

[22] Welford, Mark, and Brian H. Bossak. "Revisiting the Medieval Black Death of 1347–1351: Spatiotemporal Dynamics Suggestive of an Alternate Causation." Geography Compass 4.6 (2010): 561-575

[23] Baggaley, Kate (24 Feb 2015). "Bubonic plague was a serial visitor in European Middle Ages". Science News. Retrieved 24 February 2015.

[24] Schmid, Boris V. (2015). "Climate-driven introduction of the Black Death and successive plague reintroductions into Europe". *Proc National Academy of Sciences.* doi:10.1073/pnas.1412887112. Retrieved 24 February 2015.

[25] Byrne 2004, pp. 21–9

[26] Giovanni Boccaccio (1351). "Decameron".

[27] Ziegler 1998, p. 18,19.

[28] D. Herlihy, *The Black Death and the Transformation of the West* (Harvard University Press: Cambridge, Massachusetts, 1997), p. 29.

[29] Horrox, Rosemary (1994). *Black Death.* ISBN 978-0-7190-3498-5.

[30] In Homer's *Odyssey*, Scylla's mouth is said to contain rows of teeth "full of black death" (πλείοι μέλανος θανάτοιο).

[31] See: Stephen d'Irsay (May 1926) "Notes to the origin of the expression: atra mors," *Isis,* **8** (2) : 328-332.

[32] As seen in John of Fordun's *Scotichronicon*, where he writes "there was a great pestilence and mortality of men". Horrox, Rosemary (1994). *Black Death.* ISBN 978-0-7190-3498-5.

[33] J. M. Bennett and C. W. Hollister, *Medieval Europe: A Short History* (New York: McGraw-Hill, 2006), p. 326.

[34]
- On page 22 of the manuscript in Gallica, Simon mentions the phrase "*mors nigra*" (Black Death): "*Cum rex finisset oracula judiciorum / Mors nigra surrexit, et gentes reddidit illi;*" (When the king ended the oracles of judgment / Black Death arose, and the nations surrendered to him;).
- A more legible copy of the poem appears in: Emile Littré (1841) "Opuscule relatif à la peste de 1348, composé par un contemporain" (Work concerning the plague of 1348, composed by a contemporary), *Bibliothèque de l'école des chartes,* **2** (2) : 201-243; see especially page 228.
- See also: Joseph Patrick Byrne, *The Black Death* (Westport, Connecticut: Greenwood Press, 2004), page 1.

[35] Francis Aidan Gasquet, *The Black Death of 1348 and 1349,* 2nd ed. (London, England: George Bell and Sons, 1908), page 7. Johan Isaksson Pontanus, *Rerum Danicarum Historia ...* (Amsterdam (Netherlands): Johann Jansson, 1631), page 476.

[36] The German physician Justus Hecker (1795–1850) cited the phrase in Icelandic (*Svartur Daudi*), Danish (*den sorte Dod*), etc. See: J.F.C. Hecker, *Der schwarze Tod im vierzehnten Jahrhundert* [The Black Death in the Fourteenth Century] (Berlin, (Germany): Friedr. Aug. Herbig, 1832), page 3.

[37] The name "Black Death" first appeared in English in:
- "Mrs. Markham" (pen name of Elizabeth Penrose (née Cartwright)), *A History of England ...* (Edinburgh, Scotland: Archibald Constable, 1823). In the 1829 edition, the relevant text appeared on pages 249-250, where, about the English king Edward III, she wrote: "Edward's successes in France were interrupted during the next six years by a most terrible pestilence — so terrible as to be called the black death — which raged throughout Europe, and proved

a greater scourge to the people than even the calamities of war." (For further information about this book and Mrs. Penrose, see: Wikisource and the Oxford Dictionary of National Biography).

- See also: J. L. Bolton, "Looking for *Yersinia pestis*: Scientists, Historians and the Black Death" in: Linda Clark and Carole Rawcliffe, ed.s, *The Fifteenth Century XII: Society in an Age of Plague* (Woodbridge, England: Boydell Press, 2013), page 15.

The name "Black Death" was spread more widely when in 1833, Benjamin Guy Babington published an English translation of J.F.C. Hecker's book *Der schwarze Tod im vierzehnten Jahrhundert* as: J.F.C. Hecker with Benjamin Guy Babington, trans., *The Black Death in the Fourteenth Century* (London, England: A. Schloss, 1833).

[38] "Plague Backgrounder". Avma.org. Archived from the original on 16 May 2008. Retrieved 3 November 2008.

[39] Horrox 1994, p. 159.

[40] Sehdev PS (2002). "The Origin of Quarantine". *Clinical Infectious Diseases* **35** (9): 1071–1072. doi:10.1086/344062. PMID 12398064.

[41] Christakos, George; Olea, Ricardo A.; Serre, Marc L.; Yu, Hwa-Lung; Wang, Lin-Lin (2005). *Interdisciplinary Public Health Reasoning and Epidemic Modelling: the Case of Black Death*. Springer. pp. 110–14. ISBN 3-540-25794-2.

[42] Gasquet 1893.

[43] R. Totaro, *Suffering in Paradise: The Bubonic Plague in English Literature from More to Milton* (Pittsburgh: Duquesne University Press, 2005), p. 26.

[44] Byrne 2004, p. 8.

[45] Drancourt M, Aboudharam G, Signoli M, Dutour O, Raoult D (1998). "Detection of 400-year-old Yersinia pestis DNA in human dental pulp: an approach to the diagnosis of ancient septicemia". *Proc Natl Acad Sci U S A* **95** (21): 12637–12640. doi:10.1073/pnas.95.21.12637. PMC 22883. PMID 9770538. see alsoMichel Drancourt; Didier Raoult (2004). "Molecular detection of Yersinia pestis in dental pulp". *Microbiology* **150** (2): 263–264. doi:10.1099/mic.0.26885-0.

[46] Haensch S, Bianucci R, Signoli M, Rajerison M, Schultz M, Kacki S, Vermunt M, Weston DA, Hurst D, Achtman M, Carniel E, Bramanti B (2010). Besansky, Nora J, ed. "Distinct Clones of Yersinia pestis Caused the Black Death". *PLoS Pathogens* **6** (10): e1001134. doi:10.1371/journal.ppat.1001134. PMC 2951374. PMID 20949072.

[47] Schuenemann VJ, Bos K, DeWitte S, Schmedes S, Jamieson J, Mittnik A, Forrest S, Coombes BK, Wood JW, Earn DJD, White W, Krause J, Poinar H (2011): Targeted enrichment of ancient pathogens yielding the pPCP1 plasmid of Yersinia pestis from victims of the Black Death.

PNAS 2011; published ahead of print 29 August 2011, doi:10.1073/pnas.1105107108

[48] Thorpe, Vanessa (29 March 2014). "Black death was not spread by rat fleas, say researchers". *theguardian.com*. Retrieved 29 March 2014.

[49] Black Death skeletons unearthed by Crossrail project

[50] Ziegler 1998, p. 233.

[51] Walloe, Lars (2008). Vivian Nutton, ed. *Medieval and Modern Bubonic Plague: some clinical continuities*. Pestilential Complexities: Understanding Medieval Plague. Wellcome Trust Centre for the History of Medicine at UCL. p. 69.

[52] M. Kennedy. "Black Death study lets rats off the hook". *The Guardian* (London: The History Press Ltd). ISBN 0-7524-2829-2..

[53] B. Slone. *The Black Death in London*. London: The History Press Ltd. ISBN 0-7524-2829-2..

[54] Philip Daileader, *The Late Middle Ages*, audio/video course produced by The Teaching Company, (2007) ISBN 978-1-59803-345-8.

[55] Q&A by Kathryn Jean Lopez (14 September 2005). "Q&A with John Kelly on The Great Mortality on National Review Online". Nationalreview.com. Retrieved 10 December 2011.

[56] Egypt – Major Cities, *U.S. Library of Congress*

[57] Snell, Melissa (2006). "The Great Mortality". Historymedren.about.com. Retrieved 19 April 2009.

[58] Dick, HC; Pringle, JK; Sloane, B; Carver, J; Wisneiwski, KD; Haffenden, A; Porter, S; Roberts, D; Cassidy, NJ (2015). "Detection and characterisation of Black Death burials by multi-proxy geophysical methods". *Journal of Archaeological Sciences* **59**: 132–141. doi:10.1016/j.jas.2015.04.010.

[59] Richard Wunderli (1992). *Peasant Fires: The Drummer of Niklashausen*. Indiana University Press. p. 52. ISBN 0-253-36725-5.

[60] J. M. Bennett and C. W. Hollister, *Medieval Europe: A Short History* (New York: McGraw-Hill, 2006), p. 329.

[61] David Nirenberg, *Communities of Violence*, 1998, ISBN 0-691-05889-X.

[62] R.I. Moore *The Formation of a Persecuting Society*, Oxford, 1987 ISBN 0-631-17145-2

[63] Black Death, Jewishencyclopedia.com

[64] "Jewish History 1340–1349".

[65] "*The Great Plague*". Stephen Porter (2009). Amberley Publishing. p.25. ISBN 1-84868-087-2

[66] J. N. Hays (1998). *"The burdens of disease: epidemics and human response in western history.".* p 58. ISBN 0-8135-2528-4

[67] *"Epidemics and pandemics: their impacts on human history".* J. N. Hays (2005). p.46. ISBN 1-85109-658-2

[68] Geoffrey Parker (2001). *"Europe in crisis, 1598–1648".* Wiley-Blackwell. p.7. ISBN 0-631-22028-3

[69] *The Black Death in Egypt and England: A Comparative Study,* Stuart J. Borsch, Austin: University of Texas

[70] Secondary sources such as the *Cambridge History of Medieval England* often contain discussions of methodology in reaching these figures that are necessary reading for anyone wishing to understand this controversial episode in more detail.

[71] "BBC – History – Black Death". BBC. p. 131. Retrieved 3 November 2008.

[72] Gottfried, Robert S. (1983). *The Black Death: Natural and Human Disaster in Medieval Europe.* London: Hale. ISBN 0-7090-1299-3.

[73] "BBC – Radio 4 Voices of the Powerless – 29 August 2002 Plague in Tudor and Stuart Britain". BBC. Retrieved 3 November 2008.

[74] Plague, 1911 Edition of the Encyclopædia Britannica

[75] Vanessa Harding (2002). *"The dead and the living in Paris and London, 1500–1670.".* p.25. ISBN 0-521-81126-0

[76] Byrne 2004, p. 62.

[77] Vanessa Harding (2002). *"The dead and the living in Paris and London, 1500–1670.".* p.24. ISBN 0-521-81126-0

[78] "Plague in London: spatial and temporal aspects of mortality", J. A. I. Champion, *Epidemic Disease in London, Centre for Metropolitan History Working Papers Series,* No. 1 (1993).

[79] Geography, climate, population, economy, society. J.P.Sommerville.

[80] *"Crisis and Change in the Venetian Economy in the Sixteenth and Seventeenth Centuries".* Brian Pullan. (2006). p.151. ISBN 0-415-37700-5

[81] *"Medicine and society in early modern Europe".* Mary Lindemann (1999). Cambridge University Press. p.41. ISBN 0-521-42354-6

[82] Harald Aastorp (1 August 2004). "Svartedauden enda verre enn antatt". Forskning.no. Retrieved 3 January 2009.

[83] Øivind Larsen. "DNMS.NO : Michael: 2005 : 03/2005 : Book review: Black Death and hard facts". Dnms.no. Retrieved 3 November 2008.

[84] Karl Julius Beloch, *Bevölkerungsgeschichte Italiens,* volume 3, pp. 359–360.

[85] "Naples in the 1600s". Faculty.ed.umuc.edu. Retrieved 3 November 2008.

[86] The Seventeenth-Century Decline, S. G. Payne, *A History of Spain and Portugal*

[87] *"Armies of pestilence: the effects of pandemics on history".* James Clarke & Co. (2004). p.72. ISBN 0-227-17240-X

[88] "Kathy McDonough, Empire of Poland". Depts.washington.edu. Retrieved 3 November 2008.

[89] *"Bubonic plague in early modern Russia: public health and urban disaster".* John T. Alexander (2002). Oxford University Press US. p.21. ISBN 0-19-515818-0

[90] "Ruttopuisto – Plague Park". Tabblo.com. Retrieved 3 November 2008.

[91] *"Stockholm: A Cultural History".* Tony Griffiths (2009). Oxford University Press US. p.9. ISBN 0-19-538638-8

[92] "The Islamic World to 1600: The Mongol Invasions (The Black Death)". Ucalgary.ca. Retrieved 10 December 2011.

[93] Byrne, Joseph Patrick (2008). *Encyclopedia of Pestilence, Pandemics, and Plagues: A-M.* ABC-CLIO. p. 519. ISBN 0-313-34102-8.

[94] *"Christian Slaves, Muslim Masters: White Slavery in the Mediterranean, the Barbary Coast and Italy, 1500–1800".* Robert Davis (2004) ISBN 1-4039-4551-9.

[95] Université de Strasbourg. Institut de turcologie, Université de Strasbourg. Institut d'études turques, Association pour le développement des études turques. (1998). *Turcica.* Éditions Klincksieck. p. 198.

[96] *"The Fertile Crescent, 1800–1914: a documentary economic history".* Charles Philip Issawi (1988). Oxford University Press US. p.99. ISBN 0-19-504951-9

[97] Infectious Diseases: Plague Through History, sciencemag.org

[98] Bubonic Plague comes to Sydney in 1900, University of Sydney, Sydney Medical School

[99] Chase, Marilyn (2004). *The Barbary Plague: The Black Death in Victorian San Francisco.* Random House Digital. ISBN 0-375-75708-2.
Echenberg, Myron (2007). *Plague Ports: The Global Urban Impact of Bubonic Plague: 1894–1901.* Sacramento: New York University Press. ISBN 0-8147-2232-6.
Kraut, Alan M. (1995). *Silent travelers: germs, genes, and the "immigrant menace".* JHU Press. ISBN 0-8018-5096-7.
Markel, Howard (2005). *When Germs Travel: Six Major Epidemics That Have Invaded America And the Fears They Have Unleashed.* Random House Digital. ISBN 0-375-72602-0.
Kalisch, Philip A. (Summer 1972). "The Black Death in Chinatown: Plague and Politics in San Francisco 1900–1904". *Arizona and the West* (Journal of the Southwest) **14**

(2): 113–136. JSTOR 40168068.

Risse, Guenter B. (2012). "Bubonic Plague Visits San Francisco's Chinatown". *Plague, Fear, and Politics in San Francisco's Chinatown*. JHU Press. ISBN 1-4214-0510-5.

Shah, Nayan (2001). *Contagious divides: Epidemics and race in San Francisco's Chinatown*. University of California Press. ISBN 0-520-22629-1.

[100] Human Plague – United States, 1993–1994, Centers for Disease Control and Prevention

[101] Madon MB, Hitchcock JC, Davis RM, Myers CM, Smith CR, Fritz CL, Emery KW, O'Rullian W (1997). "An overview of plague in the United States and a report of investigations of two human cases in Kern county, California, 1995". *Journal of vector ecology : journal of the Society for Vector Ecology* **22** (1): 77–82. PMID 9221742.

[102] "Oregon man suffering from the plague is in critical condition". *Daily News* (New York). 12 June 2012.

[103] Oregon Man to Lose Fingers From Black Plague, 'Lucky' to Be Alive

[104] Drug-resistant plague a 'major threat', say scientists, SciDev.Net.

[105] "Plague - Madagascar". World Health Organisation. 21 November 2014. Retrieved 26 November 2014.

2.1.9 Further reading

- Benedictow, Ole Jørgen (2004). *Black Death 1346–1353: The Complete History*. ISBN 978-1-84383-214-0.

- Byrne, J. P. (2004). *The Black Death*. London: Greenwood Publishing Group. ISBN 0-313-32492-1.

- Cantor, Norman F. (2001), *In the Wake of the Plague: The Black Death and the World It Made*, New York, Free Press.

- Cohn, Samuel K. Jr., (2002), *The Black Death Transformed: Disease and Culture in Early Renaissance Europe*, London: Arnold.

- Gasquet, Francis Aidan (1893). *The Great Pestilence AD 1348 to 1349: Now Commonly Known As the Black Death*. ISBN 978-1-4179-7113-8.

- Hecker, J.F.C. (1859). B.G. Babington(trans), ed. *Epidemics of the Middle Ages*. London, Trübner.

- Herlihy, D., (1997), *The Black Death and the Transformation of the West*, Cambridge, Massachusetts: Harvard University Press.

- McNeill, William H. (1976). *Plagues and Peoples*. Anchor/Doubleday. ISBN 0-385-11256-4.

- Scott, S., and Duncan, C. J., (2001), *Biology of Plagues: Evidence from Historical Populations*, Cambridge: Cambridge University Press.

- Shrewsbury, J. F. D., (1970), *A History of Bubonic Plague in the British Isles*, London: Cambridge University Press

- Twigg, G., (1984), *The Black Death: A Biological Reappraisal*, London: Batsford.

- Ziegler, Philip (1998). *The Black Death*. Penguin Books. ISBN 978-0-14-027524-7. 1st editions 1969.

2.1.10 External links

-
- Black Death on *In Our Time* at the BBC. (listen now)
- Black Death at BBC

2.2 Bubonic plague

This article is about the disease in general. For information about the medieval European plague, see Black Death.

Bubonic plague is one of three types of bacterial infection caused by *Yersinia pestis*.[1] Three to seven days after exposure to the bacteria flu like symptoms develop. This includes fever, headaches, and vomiting.[1] Swollen and painful lymph nodes occur in the area closest to where the bacteria entered the skin.[2] Occasionally the swollen lymph nodes may break open.[1]

The three types of plague are the result of the route of infection: bubonic plague, septicemic plague, and pneumonic plague. Bubonic plague is mainly spread by infected fleas from small animals.[1] It may also result from exposure to the body fluids from a dead plague infected animal.[3] In the bubonic form of plague, the bacteria enter through the skin through a flea bite and travels via the lymphatic vessels to a lymph node, causing it to swell. Diagnosis is by finding the bacteria in the blood, sputum, or fluid from lymph nodes.[1]

Prevention is through public health measures such as not handling dead animals in areas where plague is common. Vaccines have not been found to be very useful for plague prevention.[1] Several antibiotics are effective for treatment including streptomycin, gentamicin, or doxycycline.[4][5] Without treatment it results in the death of 30% to 90% of those infected.[1][4] Death if it occurs is typically within ten days.[6] With treatment the risk of death is around 10%.[4] Globally in 2013 there were about 750 documented cases which resulted in 126 deaths.[1] The disease is most common in Africa.[1]

Plague is believed to be the cause of the Black Death that swept through Asia, Europe, and Africa in the 14th century and killed an estimated 50 million people.[1] This was about 25% to 60% of the European population.[1][7] Because the plague killed so many of the working population, wages rose due to the demand for labor. Some historians see this as a turning point in European economic development.[7] The term *bubonic plague* is derived from the Greek word βουβών, meaning "groin".[8]

2.2.1 Signs and symptoms

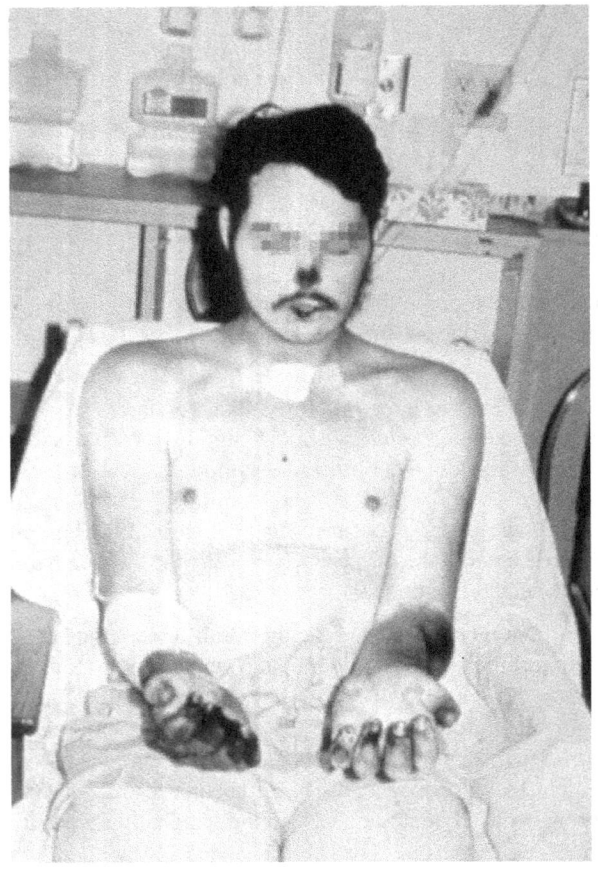

Acral necrosis of the nose, the lips, and the fingers and residual ecchymoses over both forearms in a patient recovering from bubonic plague that disseminated to the blood and the lungs. At one time, the patient's entire body was ecchymotic. Reprinted from Textbook of Military Medicine.

The best-known symptom of bubonic plague is one or more infected, enlarged, and painful lymph nodes, known as buboes. After being transmitted via the bite of an infected flea, the *Y. pestis* bacteria become localized in an inflamed lymph node where they begin to colonize and reproduce. Buboes associated with the bubonic plague are commonly found in the armpits, upper femoral, groin and neck region. Acral gangrene (i.e., of the fingers, toes, lips and nose) is another common symptom.

Because of its bite-based mode of transmission, the bubonic plague is often the first of a progressive series of illnesses. Bubonic plague symptoms appear suddenly a few days after exposure to the bacterium. Symptoms include:

- Chills
- General ill feeling (malaise)
- High fever (39 °C; 102 °F)
- Muscle cramps[9]
- Seizures
- Smooth, painful lymph gland swelling called a bubo, commonly found in the groin, but may occur in the armpits or neck, most often near the site of the initial infection (bite or scratch)
- Pain may occur in the area before the swelling appears
- Gangrene of the extremities such as toes, fingers, lips and tip of the nose.[10]

Other symptoms include heavy breathing, continuous vomiting of blood (hematemesis), aching limbs, coughing, and extreme pain caused by the decay or decomposition of the skin while the person is still alive. Additional symptoms include extreme fatigue, gastrointestinal problems, lenticulae (black dots scattered throughout the body), delirium, and coma.

2.2.2 Cause

Bubonic plague is an infection of the lymphatic system, usually resulting from the bite of an infected flea, *Xenopsylla cheopis* (the rat flea). In very rare circumstances, as in the septicemic plague, the disease can be transmitted by direct contact with infected tissue or exposure to the cough of another human. The flea is parasitic on house and field rats, and seeks out other prey when its rodent hosts die. The bacteria remained harmless to the flea, allowing the new host to spread the bacteria. The bacteria form aggregates in the gut of infected fleas and this results in the flea regurgitating ingested blood, which is now infected, into the bite site of a rodent or human host. Once established, bacteria rapidly spread to the lymph nodes and multiply.

Y. pestis bacilli can resist phagocytosis and even reproduce inside phagocytes and kill them. As the disease progresses,

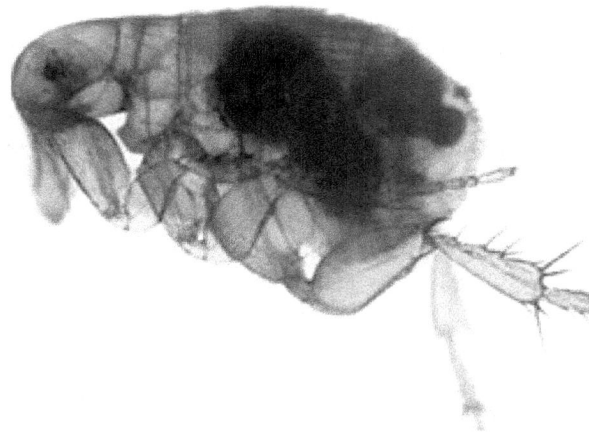

*Oriental rat flea (*Xenopsylla cheopis*) infected with the* Yersinia pestis *bacterium which appears as a dark mass in the gut. The foregut of this flea is blocked by a* Y. pestis *biofilm; when the flea attempts to feed on an uninfected host,* Y. pestis *from the foregut is regurgitated into the wound, causing infection.*

the lymph nodes can haemorrhage and become swollen and necrotic. Bubonic plague can progress to lethal septicemic plague in some cases. The plague is also known to spread to the lungs and become the disease known as the pneumonic plague.

2.2.3   Diagnosis

Laboratory testing is required in order to diagnose and confirm plague. Ideally, confirmation is through the identification of *Y. pestis* culture from a patient sample. Confirmation of infection can be done by examining serum taken during the early and late stages of infection. To quickly screen for the *Y. pestis* antigen in patients, rapid dipstick tests have been developed for field use.[11]

2.2.4   Treatment

Several classes of antibiotics are effective in treating bubonic plague. These include aminoglycosides such as streptomycin and gentamicin, tetracyclines (especially doxycycline), and the fluoroquinolone ciprofloxacin. Mortality associated with treated cases of bubonic plague is about 1–15%, compared to a mortality of 40–60% in untreated cases.[12]

People potentially infected with the plague need immediate treatment and should be given antibiotics within 24 hours of the first symptoms to prevent death. Other treatments include oxygen, intravenous fluids, and respiratory support. People who have had contact with anyone infected by pneumonic plague are given prophylactic antibiotics.[13] Using

the broad-based antibiotic streptomycin has proven to be dramatically successful against the bubonic plague within 12 hours of infection.[14]

2.2.5   History

First outbreak

Main article: Plague of Justinian

The first recorded epidemic affected the Eastern Roman Empire (Byzantine Empire) and was named the Plague of Justinian after emperor Justinian I, who was infected but survived through extensive treatment.[15][16] The pandemic resulted in the deaths of an estimated 25 million (6th century outbreak) to 50 million people (two centuries of recurrence).[17][18] The historian Procopius wrote, in Volume II of History of the Wars, of his personal encounter with the plague and the effect it had on the rising empire. In the spring of 542, the plague arrived in Constantinople, working its way from port city to port city and spreading around the Mediterranean Sea, later migrating inland eastward into Asia Minor and west into Greece and Italy. Because the infectious disease spread inland by the transferring of merchandise through Justinian's efforts in acquiring luxurious goods of the time and exporting supplies, his capital became the leading exporter of the bubonic plague. Procopius, in his work *Secret History*, declared that Justinian was a demon of an emperor who either created the plague himself or was being punished for his sinfulness.[18]

Second outbreak

Main articles: Black Death and Second plague pandemic

In the Late Middle Ages (1340–1400) Europe experienced the most deadly disease outbreak in history when the Black Death, the infamous pandemic of bubonic plague, hit in 1347, killing a third of the human population. It is believed that society subsequently became more violent as the mass mortality rate cheapened life and thus increased warfare, crime, popular revolt, waves of flagellants, and persecution.[19] The Black Death originated in or near China and spread from Italy and then throughout other European countries. Arab historians Ibn Al-Wardni and Al-maqrizi believed the Black Death originated in Mongolia, and this was proven correct as Chinese records showed a huge outbreak in Mongolia in the early 1330s.[20] Research published in 2002 suggests that it began in early 1346 in the steppe region, where a plague reservoir stretches from the northwestern shore of the Caspian Sea into southern Russia. The Mongols had cut off the trade route, the Silk Road, between China and Europe which halted the spread of the

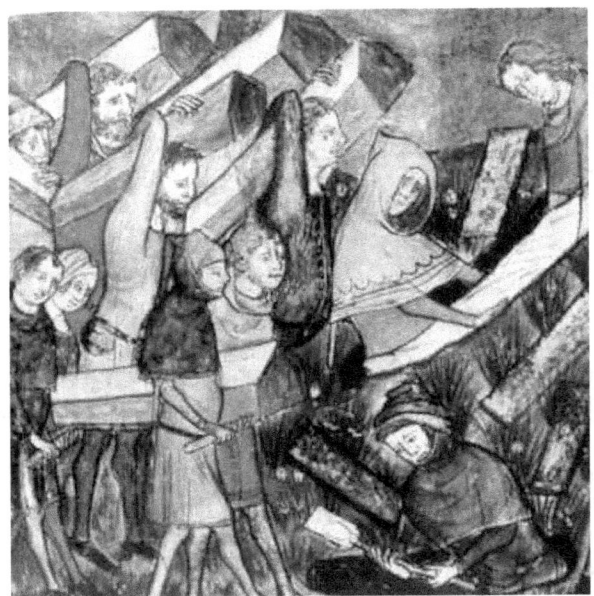

Citizens of Tournai bury plague victims. Miniature from The Chronicles of Gilles Li Muisis *(1272–1352). Bibliothèque royale de Belgique, MS 13076-77, f. 24v.*

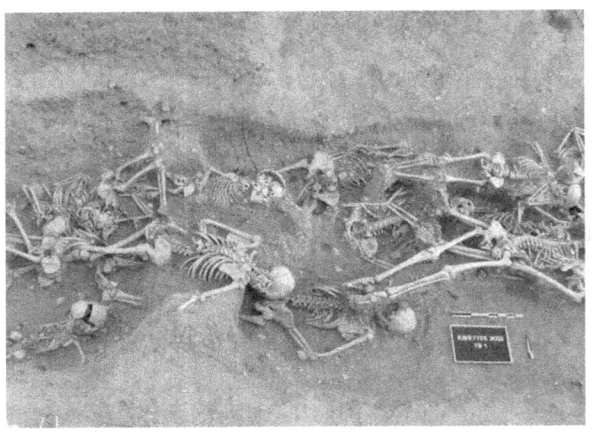

Bubonic plague victims in a mass grave from 1720–1721 in Martigues, France

Black Death from eastern Russia to Western Europe. The epidemic began with an attack that Mongols launched on the Italian merchants' last trading station in the region, Caffa in the Crimea.[14] In late 1346, plague broke out among the besiegers and from them penetrated into the town. When spring arrived, the Italian merchants fled on their ships, unknowingly carrying the Black Death. Carried by the fleas on rats, the plague initially spread to humans near the Black Sea and then outwards to the rest of Europe as a result of people fleeing from one area to another.

There were many ethno-medical beliefs for avoiding the Black Death. One of the most famous was that by walking around with flowers in or around their nose people would be able to "ward off the stench and perhaps the evil that afflicted them". People believed the plague to be a punishment from God, and that the only way to be rid of the plague was to be forgiven by God.[21] One such method used was to carve the symbol of the cross onto the front door of a house with the words "Lord have mercy on us".[22]

Pistoia, a city in Italy, went as far as enacting rules and regulations on the city and its inhabitants to keep it safe from the Black Death. The rules stated that no one was allowed to visit any plague-infected area and if they did they were not allowed back into the city. Some other rules were that no linen or woollen goods were to be imported into the city and no corpses were to be buried in the city. Despite strict enforcement of the rules, the city eventually became infected.[23] People who were not infected with the plague gathered in groups and stayed away from the sick. They ate and drank with limited food and water and were not even allowed oral communication because merely talking with one another increased the chance of passing on the disease.[24]

While Europe was devastated by the disease, the rest of the world fared much better. In India, population rose from a population of 91 million in 1300, to 97 million in 1400, to 105 million in 1500. Sub-Saharan Africa remained largely unaffected by the plagues.[25]

The next few centuries were marked by several localized or regional outbreaks of lesser severity. The Great Plague of Milan (1629-1631), the Great Plague of Seville (1647), the Great Plague of London (1665–1666), the Great Plague of Vienna (1679), Great Baltic plague (1708–1712) and the Great Plague of Marseille (1720), were the last major outbreaks of the bubonic plague in Europe.

Traditional treatment

Main article: Miasma theory

Medieval doctors thought the plague was created by air corrupted by humid weather, decaying unburied bodies, and fumes produced by poor sanitation. The recommended treatment of the plague was a good diet, rest, and relocating to a non-infected environment so the individual could get access to clean air. This did help, but not for the reasons the doctors of the time thought. In actuality, because they recommended moving away from unsanitary conditions, people were, in effect, getting away from the rodents that harbored the fleas carrying the infection. However, this also helped to spread the infection to new areas previously non-infected.

Third outbreak

Main article: Third plague pandemic
The plague resurfaced for a third time in the mid-19th cen-

DIRECTIONS FOR SEARCHERS.

1.—A search party is composed of three British soldiers and a Native gentleman. It is provided with a pickaxe, a lantern, a pot of paint and a note-book.

2.—A search division is composed of 10 search parties and is under the command of an officer. A Medical Officer, one or more ladies and three Native soldiers are attached to each search division. It is provided with two ambulances and one cart to convey property to the segregation camp.

3.—Search parties will make careful house-to-house inspection in the area assigned to their division in order to discover plague cases and dead bodies.

4.—When a search party comes to a house, the Native gentlemen will explain the object of the visit to the inmates and demand admission.

5.—Should the inmates fail to admit the search party promptly or should there be no one to open the house door the search party will force their way in.

6.—The soldiers will carefully search all parts of the house, and in doing so may force open all inner doors which are not on application opened by the inmates.

7.—In the case of the house of a Hindu the soldiers will not enter the cook-room or the god room unless—

(i) There are persons in these rooms who refuse to leave them, or
(ii) There is reason to suspect that these rooms contain a corpse or a sick person, or
(iii) Access to other portions of the house can only be obtained through these rooms.

8.—The soldiers will inspect all persons in the house in order to ascertain whether any of them are sick, provided that if the inmates so desire the inspection of the women in the house will be made by one of the ladies attached to the division.

9.—It is the duty of the Native gentlemen attached to a search party to accompany the party through the house, to act as interpreter between the soldiers and the inmates of the house, to point out to them the god rooms and the cook-room, to search these rooms himself in cases in which there is no religious objection to his doing so, and to obey the orders given to him by the officer commanding the division.

10.—The soldiers will not open boxes or cupboards unless they have reason to suspect that they contain corpses or sick persons.

11.—On a corpse or a sick person being found one member of the party will summon the Medical Officer attached to the division, while the remainder will detain the inmates of the house. Should the Medical Officer after examination suspect that the case is one of plague a segregation squad will be sent for. Any person that the Medical Officer suspects to be suffering from plague will be removed in an ambulance with one member of the household as an attendant (should any be willing to accompany him) to a plague hospital. Such of the remaining inmates of the house as the Medical Officer may indicate will be taken charge of by the segregation squad. The inmates of the house and the neighbours should be desired to make immediate arrangements for the burial or burning of any corpse that may be found. Should nobody be found willing to undertake this duty a funeral party will be summoned from the City Police office.

12.—The officer in charge of a search division will note the names of all plague patients and corpses and the number of the house, name of Street and the Peth where the patients and corpses are found.

13.—The inmates of any infected house which is ordered to be vacated will be required to choose whether such valuable property as they may possess should be delivered to a neighbour after disinfection or should be sent to the warehouse. If they chose the latter alternative the property will be packed and marked with the letter W.

14.—Persons removed to a plague hospital may take with them only such articles as the Medical Officer may permit. Persons removed to a segregation camp may send to the camp clothes, bedding, cooking pots and other necessaries and comforts in the cart assigned for that purpose.

15. Except property to be removed to a plague hospital or a segregation camp no property shall be removed from an infected house till the house has been disinfected by the fumigators.

16.—The mat or bedding of a plague patient will be burnt in the street, but no other property will be destroyed by search parties.

17 After searching a house the search party will paint such mark upon it as may from time to time be prescribed as a sign that it has been searched. An account must be kept of the number of houses searched.

18 The Medical Officer will cause a vertical red line to be painted on each infected house and the date of search to be painted beside it.

19.—The Native soldiers attached to a search division will be employed on fastening up doors that have been forced open.

20 The Medical Officer will be accompanied by a man carrying a yellow flag to show his whereabouts.

Directions for searchers, Poona (now Pune) plague of 1897

tury. Like the two previous outbreaks, this one also originated in Eastern Asia.[26] The initial outbreak occurred in China's Yunnan province in 1855.[27] The disease remained localized in Southwest China for several years before spreading. In the city of Canton, beginning in March 1894, the disease killed 60,000 people in a few weeks. Daily water-traffic with the nearby city of Hong Kong rapidly spread the plague there, killing over 100,000 within two months.[28]

From China, the plague spread to the Indian subcontinent around 1896. Over the next thirty years, India would lose 12.5 million people to the bubonic plague. The disease was initially seen in port cities, beginning with Bombay (now Mumbai), but later emerged in Poona (now Pune),

Kolkata, and Karachi (now in Pakistan). By 1899, the outbreak spread to smaller communities and rural areas in many regions of India. Overall, the impact of plague epidemics was greatest in western and northern India—in the provinces then designated as Bombay, Punjab, and the United Provinces—while eastern and southern India were not as badly affected. Ultimately, more than 12 million people died from the plague in India (including present day Pakistan and Bangladesh) and China alone.

In 1899, the plague reached the islands of Hawaii.[29] The first evidence of the disease was found in Honolulu's Chinatown on Oahu.[30] It was located very close to the island's piers, and rats in cargo ships from China were able to land on the Hawaiian islands unseen. As the rats, hosts for disease-carrying fleas, made their way deeper into the city, people started to fall ill. On December 12, 1899, the first case was confirmed. The Board of Health then quickly thought of ways to prevent the disease from spreading even further inland. Their solution was to burn down any buildings in Chinatown suspected of containing a source of the disease. On December 31, 1899, the board set the first fire. They had originally planned to burn only a few targeted buildings, and thought they could control the flames as each building was finished, but the fire got out of control, burning down untargeted neighboring buildings. The resulting fire caused many of Chinatown's homes to be destroyed and an estimated 4,000 people were left homeless.[31]

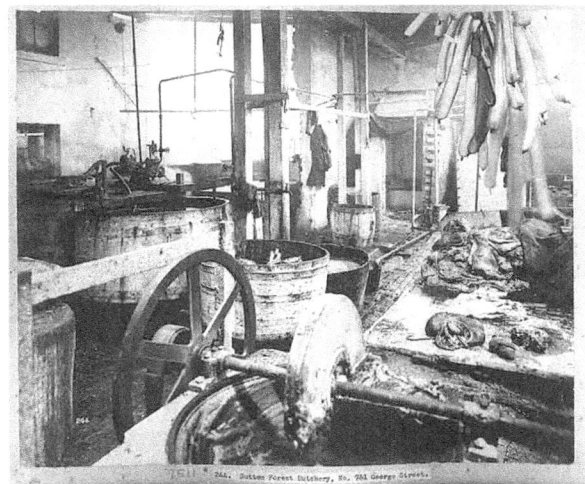

From a series of images depicting the state of houses and "slum" buildings in Sydney, Australia at the time of the 1900 outbreak and the cleansing and disinfecting operations which followed.

Australia suffered 12 major plague outbreaks between 1900 and 1925 originating from shipping.[32] Research by Australian medical officers Thompson, Armstrong and Tidswell contributed to understanding the spread of *Yersinia pestis* to humans by fleas from infected rats.[33]

According to the World Health Organization, the pandemic was considered active until 1959, when worldwide casualties dropped to 200 per year. In 1994, a plague outbreak in five Indian states caused an estimated 700 infections (including 52 deaths) and triggered a large migration of Indians within India as they tried to avoid the plague.

2.2.6 Biological warfare

Some of the earliest instances of biological warfare were said to have been products of the plague, as armies of the 14th century were recorded catapulting diseased corpses over the walls of towns and villages to spread the pestilence.

Later, plague was used during the Second Sino-Japanese War as a bacteriological weapon by the Imperial Japanese Army. These weapons were provided by Shirō Ishii's units and used in experiments on humans before being used on the field. For example, in 1940, the Imperial Japanese Army Air Service bombed Ningbo with fleas carrying the bubonic plague.[34] During the Khabarovsk War Crime Trials, the accused, such as Major General Kiyashi Kawashima, testified that, in 1941, some 40 members of Unit 731 air-dropped plague-contaminated fleas on Changde. These operations caused epidemic plague outbreaks.[35]

2.2.7 See also

- List of cutaneous conditions
- List of epidemics
- Miasma theory
- Plague (disease)
- Plague doctor
- Plague doctor costume

2.2.8 Footnotes

[1] World Health Organization (November 2014). "Plague Fact sheet N°267". Retrieved 10 May 2015.

[2] "Plague Symptoms". Jun 13, 2012. Retrieved Aug 21,15. Check date values in: |access-date= (help)

[3] "Plague Ecology and Transmission". Jun 13, 2012. Retrieved Aug 21,15. Check date values in: |access-date= (help)

[4] Prentice MB, Rahalison L (2007). "Plague". *Lancet* **369** (9568): 1196–207. doi:10.1016/S0140-6736(07)60566-2. PMID 17416264.

[5] "Plague Resources for Clinicians". Jun 13, 2012. Retrieved Aug 21,15. Check date values in: |access-date= (help)

[6] Keyes, Daniel C. (2005). *Medical response to terrorism : preparedness and clinical practice*. Philadelphia [u.a.]: Lippincott Williams & Wilkins. p. 74. ISBN 9780781749862.

[7] "Plague History". Jun 13, 2012. Retrieved Aug 21,15. Check date values in: |access-date= (help)

[8] LeRoux, Neil (2007). *Martin Luther As Comforter: Writings on Death Volume 133 of Studies in the History of Christian Traditions*. BRILL. p. 247. ISBN 9789004158801.

[9] "Symptoms of Plague". *Brief Overview of Plague*. Healthagen, LLC. Retrieved November 26, 2014.

[10] Inglesby TV, Dennis DT, Henderson DA; et al. (May 2000). "Plague as a biological weapon: medical and public health management. Working Group on Civilian Biodefense". *JAMA* **283** (17): 2281–90. doi:10.1001/jama.283.17.2281. PMID 10807389.

[11] "Plague, Laboratory testing". *Health Topics A to Z*. Retrieved 23 October 2010.

[12] "Plague". Retrieved 25 February 2010.

[13] "Plague". Healthagen, LLC. Retrieved 4 April 2011.

[14] Echenberg,Myron (2002). Pestis Redux: The Initial Years of the Third Bubonic Plague Pandemic, 1894–1901. Journal of World History,vol 13,2

[15] Little (2007), pp. 8–15.

[16] McCormick (2007), pp. 290–312.

[17] Rosen, William (2007), *Justinian's Flea: Plague, Empire, and the Birth of Europe*. Viking Adult; pg 3; ISBN 978-0-670-03855-8.

[18] Moorshead Magazines, Limited. "The Plague Of Justinian." History Magazine 11.1 (2009): 9–12. History Reference Center

[19] Cohn, Samuel K.(2002). The Black Death: End of a Paradigm. American Historical Review, vol 107, 3, pg. 703–737

[20] Sean Martin (2001). *Black Death:Chapter One*. Harpenden,GBR:Pocket Essentials. p. 14.

[21] "The Black Death". history.com. 2013. Retrieved 2013-11-14.

[22] "Mee Jr, Charles L. (2011). "The Black Death, a bubonic plague of great dimensions-part 2." Word Focus". Wordfocus.com. Retrieved 2012-12-18.

[23] "Mee Jr., Charles L. "The Black Death, a Bubonic Plague of Great Dimensions – Part 2 | WordFocus.com." Wordfocus.com | English Vocabulary Words Derived from Latin and Greek Prefixes | Etymology. Web. 02 Dec. 2011". Wordfocus.com. Retrieved 2012-12-18.

[24] Sean Martin (2001). *Black Death: Chapter Two*. Harpenden, GBR:Pocket Essentials. p. 26.

[25] Reaching Out: Expanding Horizons of Cross-Cultural Interaction

[26] Nicholas Wade (October 31, 2010). "Europe's Plagues Came From China, Study Finds". *The New York Times*. Retrieved 2010-11-01. The great waves of plague that twice devastated Europe and changed the course of history had their origins in China, a team of medical geneticists reported Sunday, as did a third plague outbreak that struck less harmfully in the 19th century.

[27] Cohn, Samuel K. (2003). *The Black Death Transformed: Disease and Culture in Early Renaissance Europe*. A Hodder Arnold. p. 336. ISBN 0-340-70646-5.

[28] Pryor, E. G. (1975). "The Great Plague OF Hong Kong" (PDF). *Journal of the Royal Asiatic Society Hong Kong Branch* (Hong Kong: Royal Asiatic Society of Great Britain and Ireland-Hong Kong Branch) **15**: 69. ISSN 1991-7295. Retrieved June 2, 2014.

[29] "Bubonic Plague Originated in China". *DNews*.

[30] "Hawaii for Visitors, retrieved on December 6, 2011". Hawaiiforvisitors.com. Retrieved 2012-12-18.

[31] "The Honolulu Advertiser, retrieved on December 6, 2011". The.honoluluadvertiser.com. Retrieved 2012-12-18.

[32] "Bubonic Plague comes to Sydney in 1900". *Sydney Medical School – Online Museum*. University of Sydney. 2012. Retrieved 2 August 2012.

[33] Thompson, J. Ashburton (1901). "A Contribution to the Aetiology of Plague". *The Journal of Hygiene* (London) **1** (2): 153–167. doi:10.1017/S0022172400000152. PMC 2235949. PMID 20474113.

[34] "The Independent - 404". *The Independent*.

[35] Daniel Barenblatt, *A Plague upon Humanity.*, 2004, pages 220–221.

2.2.9   References

- Echenberg, Myron J. (2007). *Plague Ports: The Global Urban Impact of Bubonic Plague, 1894–1901*. New York, NY: New York University Press. ISBN 0-8147-2232-6. OCLC 70292105.

- Little, Lester K. (2007). "Life and Afterlife of the First Plague Pandemic." In: Little, Lester K. editor. (2007), *Plague and the End of Antiquity: The Pandemic of 541–750*. Cambridge University Press. (2007). ISBN 978-0-521-84639-4 (hardback); ISBN 978-0-521-71897-4 (paperback).

- McCormick, Michael (2007). "Toward a Molecular History of the Justinian Pandemic." In: Little, Lester K. editor. (2007), *Plague and the End of Antiquity: The Pandemic of 541–750*. Cambridge University Press. (2007). ISBN 978-0-521-84639-4 (hardback); ISBN 978-0-521-71897-4 (paperback).

- "Bubonic Plague Originated in China", Discovery News,1 November 2010. Retrieved on 6 December 2011.

- "Bubonic Plague Fire Destroyed Honolulu's Chinatown" Hawaii for Visitors. Retrieved on 6 December 2011.

- "Bubonic Plague and the Chinatown Fire Honolulu Advertiser, 7 July 2005. Retrieved on 6 December 2011.

2.2.10   Further reading

- Alexander, John T. (2003) [First published 1980]. *Bubonic Plague in Early Modern Russia: Public Health and Urban Disaster*. Oxford, UK; New York, NY: Oxford University Press. ISBN 0-19-515818-0. OCLC 50253204.

- Carol, Benedict (1996). *Bubonic Plague in Nineteenth-Century China*. Stanford, CA: Stanford University Press. ISBN 0-8047-2661-2. OCLC 34191853.

- Biddle, Wayne (2002). *A Field Guide to Germs* (2nd Anchor Books ed.). New York: Anchor Books. ISBN 1-4000-3051-X. OCLC 50154403.

- Little, Lester K. (2007). *Plague and the End of Antiquity: The Pandemic of 541–750*. New York, NY: Cambridge University Press. ISBN 978-0-521-84639-4. OCLC 65361042.

- Rosen, William (2007). *Justinian's Flea: Plague, Empire and the Birth of Europe*. London, England: Viking Penguin. ISBN 978-0-670-03855-8.

- Scott, Susan, and C. J. Duncan (2001). *Biology of Plagues: Evidence from Historical Populations*. Cambridge, UK; New York, NY: Cambridge University Press. ISBN 0-521-80150-8. OCLC 44811929.

- Batten-Hill, David (2011). *This Son of York*. Kendal, England: David Batten-Hill. ISBN 978-1-78176-094-9. OCLC http://www.tsoy.co.uk.

- Kool, J. L. (2005). "Risk of Person-to-Person Transmission of Pneumonic Plague". *Clinical Infectious Diseases* **40** (8): 1166–1172. doi:10.1086/428617. PMID 15791518.

2.3 Dalhana

Dalhana was a medieval commentator on the Sushruta Samhita, an early text on Indian medicine. Dalhana's commentary is known as the ***Nibandha Samgraha***. It compiles the views of a large number of authors and commentators in the text who lived before Dalhana.

The date of Dalhana's work is determined by his quoting Cakrapani (fl. 1060) and his being quoted by Hemadri (fl. 1260), placing him between the late 11th and the early 13th century. [1]

2.3.1 References

[1] Surendranath Dasgupta. *A History of Indian Philosophy, Volume 1*. Motilal Banarsidass. p. 427.

- P. V. Sharma (1982), *Dalhana and his Comments on Drugs*, New Delhi, India Munshiram Manoharlal Publishers, ISBN 9788121501590.

- P. V. Sharma (1999), *Susruta-Samhita: With English Translation of Text and Dalhana's Commentary Along with Critical Notes*, 3 Vols. Vol. I: Sutrasthana, Vol. II: Kalpasthana and Uttaratantra, Vol. III: Nidana, Sarira and Cikitsasthana; Chowkhamba Visvabharati; Varanasi.

2.4 Hakim Syed Zillur Rahman

Hakim Syed Zillur Rahman (Urdu: حکیم سید ظل الرحمن) (Bengali: হাকিম সৈয়দ জিল্লুর রহমান), is well known for his contribution to Unani medicine. He founded Ibn Sina Academy of Medieval Medicine and Sciences in 2000. He has earlier served as Professor and chairman, Department of Ilmul Advia at the Ajmal Khan Tibbiya College, Aligarh Muslim University, Aligarh, for over 40 years before retiring as Dean Faculty of Unani Medicine.

Author of 45 books and several papers on different aspects of Unani, he also owns one of the largest collection of books on Unani medicine.

The Government of India conferred him with Padma Shri award in 2006 for his contribution in the field of Unani Medicine.[1]

2.4.1 Biography

Early life and education

Rahman was born on 1 July 1940, at Bhopal, Bhopal State (now in Madhya Pradesh) in a family of learned scholars. His grandfather Hakim Syed Karam Husain, father Hakim Syed Fazlur Rahman and uncle Hakim Syed Atiqul Qadir were famous Unani Physicians of their times at Tijara / Bhopal. He is married to Ahmadi Begum and has four children: Safia Akhtar, Syed Ziaur Rahman, Soofia Akhtar and Asifa Haneefa.

Rahman received his early education from Darul-uloom Nadwatul Ulama at Lucknow and later studied at Tibbiya College, Aligarh Muslim University, Aligarh.

Career

Rahman started his career from Ajmal Khan Tibbiya College, Aligarh Muslim University as Demonstrator in 1961 and then Lecturer from Jamia Tibbiya, Delhi, he was appointed reader in 1973 and professor in 1983. He remained Chairman of the Department of Ilmul Advia for 18 years and Dean of the Faculty of Unani Medicine, Aligarh Muslim University."[2][3]

2.4.2 Works

His entire work concerns with history of medicine particularly of medieval medicine and medicine in medieval Islam. He is himself a diligent explorer of Unani medicine for old Arabic and Persian manuscripts.

2.4.3 Selected bibliography

Following is the list of important books that he authored:[4]

- Daur Jadeed Aur Tibb, 1963.[5] (Book in Urdu on Modern times and Unani medicine)

- Tarikh llm Tashrih, 1967. (Book in Urdu on History of anatomy)

- Ilmul Amraz, 1969. (Based on Avicenna's tract on Pathology in Urdu)

- Resalah Judia, 1971. (Based on Avicenna's tested Prescriptions in Urdu)

- Tajdeed Tibb, 1972. (Book in Urdu on Unani medicine)

- Bayaz Waheedi, 1974. (Book in Urdu on Prescriptions and formulations by Hakim Abdul Waheed)

- Matab Murtaish, 1976. (Book in Urdu on Unani Formularies used by Azizi Family of Lucknow)

- Tazkerah Khandan Azizi 1978. (Book in Urdu on History of Azizi Family of Unani medicine)

- Kitabul Murakkabat 1980. (Book in Urdu on Pharmaceutical formulation of Unani medicine)

- Safvi Ahad Main Ilm Tashreeh Ka Mutala, 1983. (Book in Urdu on Studies of History of anatomy during Safavid dynasty)

- Hayat Karam Hussain, 1983.[6] (Biography of Hakim Syed Karam Husain in Urdu)

- The Azizi Family of Physicians, 1983. (Book in English on Azizi Family of Unani medicine)

- Aligarh Key Tibbi Makhtootat, 1984. (Book in Urdu on Manuscripts of Unani medicine extant in Aligarh)

- Qanoon lbn Sina Aur Uskey Shareheen wa Mutarjemeen, 1986.[7] (Based on references and translations of the works of Ibn Sina in Urdu)

- Risalah Nabidh (Edited with Facsimile), 1986. (Book in Urdu and Arabic on Nabidh by Qusta ibn Luqa)

- Tibb Firoz Shahi, 1990. (Book in Urdu on Unani medicine during Firuz Shah Tughlaq)

- Research in Ilmul Advia, 1990. (Book in English on Research in Unani Pharmacology)

- Risalah Atrilal, 1993. (Book in Arabic on Treatise on Ammi majus Linn)

- Studies in Ilmul Advia, 1994. (Book in English on Studies on Unani Pharmacology)

- Dilli aur Tibb Unani, 1995.[8] (Book in Urdu on History of Unani medicine in Delhi)

- AI-Advia al-Qalbia, 1996. (Book in Urdu on Avicenna's treatise on Cardiac drugs)

- Iran Nama, 1998. (Iran Travelogue / Travel journal in Urdu)

- Tibbi Taqdame, 2001. (Based on Prefaces written for many books of other Unani scholars in Urdu)

- Aina-e Tarikh Tibb, 2001. (Based on chapters written on History of Unani medicine in Urdu)

- Asmaul Advia, 2002 (Based on Names of Pharmaceutics in Unani medicine in Urdu)

- Maqalat Shifaul Mulk Hakim Abdul Latif, 2002 (Based on Unani articles written by Shifaul Mulk Hakim Abdul Latif in Urdu)

- Hakim Ajmal Khan, 2004 (Biography of Hakim Ajmal Khan in Urdu and Hindi)

- Persian Translation of Qanun Ibn Sina aur uskey Shirehin wa Mutarjamin, 2004 (Based on references and translations of the works of Ibn Sina in Persian)

- Safar Nama Bangladesh, 2006 (Bangladesh Travelogue / Travel journal in Urdu

- Jawami Kitab Al-Nabd Al-Saghir by Galen, 2007 (Based on Galen's treatise on arterial and venous pulse in Urdu and Arabic)

- Risalah Fi Auja Al Niqris by Qusta Ibn Luqa, 2007 (Based on Al Niqris by Qusta ibn Luqa in Urdu and Arabic)

- Ainul Hayat by Mohammad Ibn Yusuf Harawi, 2007 (Based on Ageing and senile problems by Muhammad ibn Yusuf al-Harawi in Urdu and Arabic)

- Rislah fil Nabidh, 2007 (Based on Arabic translation by Qusta ibn Luqa on Treatise of Nabidh by Rufus of Ephesus in Urdu and Arabic)

- Kitab al Anasir by Galen, 2008 (Based on al Anasir by Galen in Urdu and Arabic)

- Kitab Al Mizaj by Galen, 2008 (Based on Theory of temperament and Four humours by Galen in Urdu and Arabic)

- Kitab fi Firaq al Tibb by Galen 2008 (Based on a book fi al Firaq by Galen in Urdu and Arabic)

- Tazkira Atibba-e-Asr, 2010 (Biographies of Unani scholars of contemporary age in Urdu)

- Post Graduate Education, Research Methodology and Manuscript Studies in Unani Medicine, 2011 (Edited Book in English on Research methodology in Unani medicine)

- Ross Masud, 2011 (Book on the Biography of Ross Masood in Urdu)

- Mîzân-i Harf, 2012 (Book based on essays and chapters on the life of Syed Amin Ashraf)

2.4.4 Significant contributions

- By his personal efforts made the Department of Ilmul Advia, Ajmal Khan Tibbia College, Aligarh Muslim University, Aligarh as a center of excellence. A new building of the department with all modern facilities in the laboratories was constructed under his able guidance and chairmanship. He raised both name and fame of this department at national and international level.

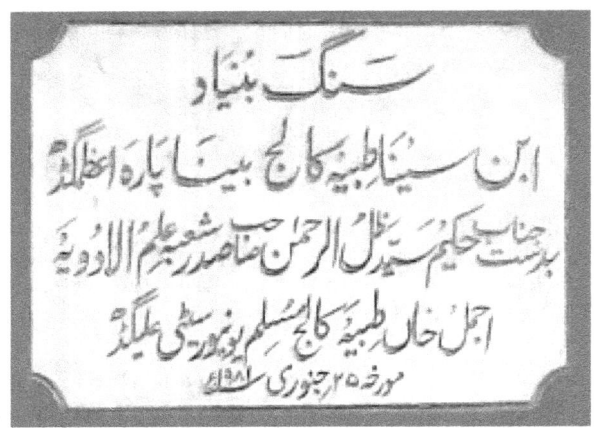

Foundation Stone, Ibn Sina Tibbiya College, Beenapara (Azamgarh)

- He assisted in the establishment of Ibn Sina Tibbia College at Beenapara, Azamgarh of which he laid the foundation stone on 25 January 1981.

- He established his personal library-cum-museum in 1960s, which became part of 'Shifa-al Mulk Hakim Abdul Latif Memorial Committee' in 1970. After the establishment of Ibn Sina Academy of Medieval Medicine and Sciences[9] in 2000, this library (Hakim Zillur Rahman Library)[10] and museum (Hakim Karam Hussain Museum on History of Medicine & Science and Hakim Fazlur Rahman Museum on Arts, Culture & Orientalism) have now become a part of the academy. The library at present houses one of the most precious and valuable collection of 20,000 printed books, 500 manuscripts",[11][12] some rare books, microfilms, compact discs, a large number of periodicals and manuscript catalogues. Books in many languages like Arabic, Persian, Urdu, Sanskrit and English on a variety of subjects like History of Medicine and History of Science, Unani, Medieval medicine, Ilmul Advia (Pharmacology), Urdu Literature with special reference to Ghalib, Iqbal, Aligarh and Sir Syed Ahmad Khan are also extant in this library. In addition, there is a Publication Division under the Shifaul

Mulk Hakim Abdul Latif Memorial Committee, Centre for Safety & Rational Use of Indian Systems of Medicine, Ibn Sina Shifakhana, AIDS Cell & Ghalib Study Centre.

- He edited 'Al-Hikmat' (Monthly Unani Literary Magazine) from 1965–1970.

2.4.5 Awards and honours

Rahman was appointed honorary visiting professor at Hamdard University in 1997 and have further been awarded the honorary degree of Doctor of Letters at a graduation ceremony in 2013.

- Ayurvedic and Tibbi Academy Award, Government of UP, Lucknow, 1968.

- Urdu Academy Award, Government of UP, Lucknow, 1974.

- Urdu Academy Award, Government of UP, Lucknow, 1978.

- Urdu Academy Award, Government of UP, Lucknow, 1993.

- Certificate of honours for outstanding contribution to Persian Language, (President of India Award on Independence day, 15 August 1995).

- Short-term Consultant, World Health Organization to the South East Asia Region for development of Unani Medicine in Bangladesh, 1996.

- Shifaul Mulk Hakim Habibur Rahman Memorial Foundation Shield, Dhaka, Bangladesh, 1996.

- Visiting Professor, Hamdard University, Karachi, Pakistan, 1997.

- Imtiaz-e Mir Award, All India Mir Academy, Lucknow, 1997.

- Pakistan Tibbi Pharmaceutical Manufacture's Council, Pakistan, 1997.

- Conferment of title: Reflective thinker and Researcher, Idara Sada-e-Qasmi, Karachi, Pakistan, 1997.

- Urdu Academy Award, Government of UP, Lucknow, 1998.

- Hakim Said Memorial Lecture, Hamdard Foundation, Hamdard University, Karachi, 2004

- Institute of Alternative Medicine, Karachi, Pakistan, 2004

- Padma Shri by Government of India, 2006.

- Ibn Sina Award, All India Unani Tibbi Congress, 2009

- Maulana Azad National Award, Milli Educational Foundation & All India Urdu Educational Committee, 2009

- Felicitated by Azam Tibbia College, Hyderabad, Sindh, Pakistan, 2004; Punjab Tibbia College, Jhang, Pakistan, 1997; Ajmal Tibbia College, Rawalpindi, Pakistan, 1997; AR Memorial Tibbia College, Lahore, Pakistan, 1997; Anjuman Himayat Islam Tibbia College, Lahore 1997, 2004 and 2008

- Hakim Ahmed Ashraf Memorial Global Award – Awarded in 2009, by Hakim Ahmed Ashraf Memorial Society (Regd.), Hyderabad.

- D.Litt (Honoris Causa) Awarded by Hamdard University, Karachi, Pakistan, 2013.

- Yash Bharti Samman, Government of Uttar Pradesh, 2015

2.4.6 See also

- Sources of Galen' works

- Writings of Qusta ibn Luqa

- Works on Ibn Sina

- Works on Rufus of Ephesus

- Ain al-Hayat by Muhammad ibn Yusuf al-Harawi

- Hakim Syed Zillur Rahman Library

- Hakim Ajmal Khan

- Hakim Habibur Rahman Foundation

- Dawakhana Shifaul Amraz

- Hakim Abdul Aziz

2.4.7 References

[1] "Padma Awards" (PDF). Ministry of Home Affairs, Government of India. 2015. Retrieved July 21, 2015.

[2] "Brief Biography". Germany.

[3] "Biography" (PDF). International Institute of Islamic Medicine, USA.

[4] "List of Books". Open Library.

[5] Hakim Syed Zillur Rahman (1962), *Daur-e Jadeed aur Tib*, Bhopal, India: Tibbi Academy, India

[6] Hakim Syed Zillur Rahman (1983, revised second edition 2008), *Ḥayāt-i Karam Ḥusain*, ʻAlīgaṛh: [s.n.] Check date values in: |date= (help)

[7] "Commentaries, Sources and Editions of The Canon of Medicine". Ibn Sina Academy of Medieval Medicine & Sciences.

[8] "Dilli aur Tibb-e Unani". Urdu Academy, Govt. of NCT, Delhi.

[9] "Visit of Ibn Sina Academy" (PDF). S. Moinuddin Alvi, Aligarh.

[10] "Zillur Rahman Library, India". United States National Library of Medicine, National Institute of Health.

[11] "Manuscripts Catalogues at Zillur Rahman Library". Microfilm Centre of India.

[12] "Manuscripts Libraries". Microfilm Centre of India.

2.4.8 Further reading

- Bhopal ka Maya-i naz Sapoot: Padma Shri Hakim Syed Zillur Rahman, by Kausar Siddiqi (Bhopal), Karwan-e Adab, January – March 2011, p. 10 – 16.

- Hakim Syed Zillur Rahman – Hayat wa Khidmat, Aik Jaiza, Swad-e Harf (First edition 2011), Authored by Dr. Mukhtar Shamim, Bhopal, p. 112 – 127.

- Hakim Syed Zillur Rahman – Eik Mut'ala (A monograph) by Dr. Fakhre Alam, Ibn Sina Academy, Aligarh, 2010; ISBN 978-93-8061-003-0.

- Hakim Syed Zillur Rahman – Hayat wa Khidmat (A voluminous biography), Ed. Dr. Hasan Abbas (Banaras Hindu University) & Dr. A. Latif (Aligarh Muslim University), Markaz Tahqiqat Farsi wa Urdu, Siwan (Bihar), 2005, page 604.

- Muslims in India, Ed. Ratna Sahai, Ministry of External Affairs, Govt. of India, New Delhi.

- Investiture Ceremony Brochure, Ministry of Human Resource Development, Dept. of Education, New Delhi, 10 August 1996.

- Hakim Syed Zillur Rahman Ek Mumtaz aur Yagana Sifat Tibbi Shakhsiyat by Basheer Zafar, Asrar-i Hikmat, Special Number, Lahore, 1970.

- Professor Hakim Syed Zillur Rahman, by Dr. Rais Ahmad Naumani, Qaumi Awaz, 4 December 1995, New Delhi and Rehnumi Sehat, Faisalabad, Pakistan, April 1998, pp. 9 – 15.

- Hakim Syed Zillur Rahman – Shakhsiyat aur Fan by Hakim Shafqat Azmi, Rahnuma-i Sehat, Faisalabad, Pakistan, January 1998.

- Mufakir wa Mohaqiq Tibb-i Unani – Professor Zillur Rahman ka Tarikhi Taruf by Hakim Mohd. Qasim Siddiqui, Sada-i Qasmi Procedures, Karachi, 1997.

- My Days at Aligarh, Autobiography by Prof. M. N. Farooqui, Former vice-chancellor, AMU, Aligarh, 1995.

- Hakim Syed Zillur Rahman ke Azeem Ilmi Karname by Mr. Farooq Nafey of Qaide Azam University, Islamabad, Tahzibul Akhlaq, Lahore, Pakistan, April 1997.

- Special Brochure on the Title Ceremony, Sada-i Qasmi, Karachi, Pakistan, July 1997.

- Souvenir, Hindustan Mein Tibbi Unani (Past, Present, Future), All India Unani Tibbi Conference, New Delhi, 1993.

- Dastawaiz, Urdu Academy, Govt. of U.P., Lucknow, 1983.

- Hakim Syed Zillur Rahman – Aik Ilmi Shakhsiyat by Prof. Nisar Ahmad Faruqui, Idrak, Gopalpur, Bakarganj, Siwan (Bihar), 213–216: No. 3, 2003

- Hakim Syed Zillur Rahman – Aik Maya' naz Shakhsiyat by Dr. Abdul Latif, Idrak, Gopalpur, Bakarganj, Siwan (Bihar), 217–222: No. 3, 2003

- Hakim Syed Zillur Rahman Number, Idrak (5), Gopalpur, Bakarganj, Siwan (Bihar), 2005.

- First "Professor Hakim Syed Zillur Rahman Oration" Delivered by Prof. Hakim Abdul Hannan, Dean, Faculty of Eastern Medicine, Hamdard University, Karachi, at International Integrative Medicine Conference, Karachi, Pakistan, 24–26 Nov. 2008

- Tibb-e Unani main Urdu tarjume ki rawayat aur Hakim Syed Zillur Rahman – aik tanqeedi aur tajziati muttala by Hakim Fakhre Alam, Uni-Med – Kulliyat 2007, Vol 3, No. 1: 2–11

- Aks Khama Hakim Syed Zillur Rahman by Hakim Fakhre Alam, Aligarh, 2008

2.5 Ibn Sina Academy of Medieval Medicine and Sciences

Ibn Sina Academy of Medieval Medicine and Sciences (IAMMS) (Urdu: ابن سینا اکا ڈ می آف میڈ یول میڈ یسین اینڈ

سائنسیز) is a trust registered under the Indian Trusts Act, 1882. Mohammad Hamid Ansari, former vice-chancellor of Aligarh Muslim University, Aligarh, formally inaugurated it on April 21, 2001. Department of AYUSH, Ministry of Health and Family Welfare, Government of India gave accreditation to the academy in 2004 and promoted it as 'centre of excellence' in 2008. Membership of the academy is open to anyone who has an interest in the academy's activities particularly on history of medicine and history of science. Being a charitable organization, donations to the Academy are also exempted from Income Tax under section 80G of the Income Tax Act 1961.

The founder president is Hakim Syed Zillur Rahman.

2.5.1 Aims and objectives

- To promote studies in the works of physicians and scientists — particularly Ibn Sina and his contemporaries —

- To propagate and disseminate in public interest the useful knowledge concerning medicine, philosophy, science and technology, social and preventive medical science, hygiene and environment.

- To inculcate in the masses an active interest in useful information regarding science, hygiene and medicine with its advances as well as the frontier areas of research, inventions and discoveries therein and also to make proper utilization of mass media for propagation, dissemination and transmission of the same.

- To establish dialogue between different theories concerning useful knowledge including the diverse prevalent systems of medical science, methodologies and philosophies;

- To preserve artefacts on Indian culture, heritage and sciences including history of medicine;

- To strive for bringing about adjustment, integration and synthesis and to organize / sponsor educational programmes, seminars, symposia, workshops and conferences as well as to promote academic work of all kinds in order to advance and develop the medical science.

Ibn Sina Academy is a part of signatories related to various health issues in the world.[1][2][3][4]

2.5.2 History

Ibn Sina Academy of Medieval Medicine and Sciences is an extension of **Majlis Ibn Sina**, which was formed in 1965

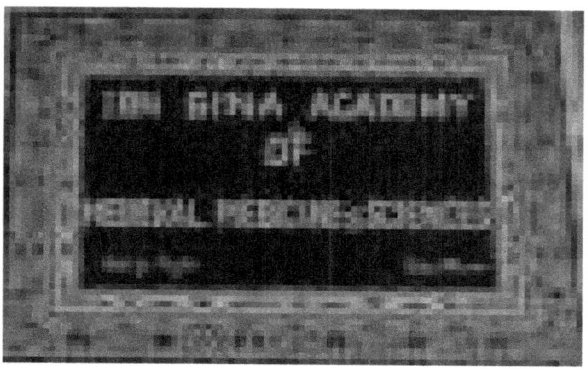

Mosaic of Iranian tiles calligraphically inscribed 'Ibn Sina Academy ...' (now destroyed during renovation; once installed at the main entrance)

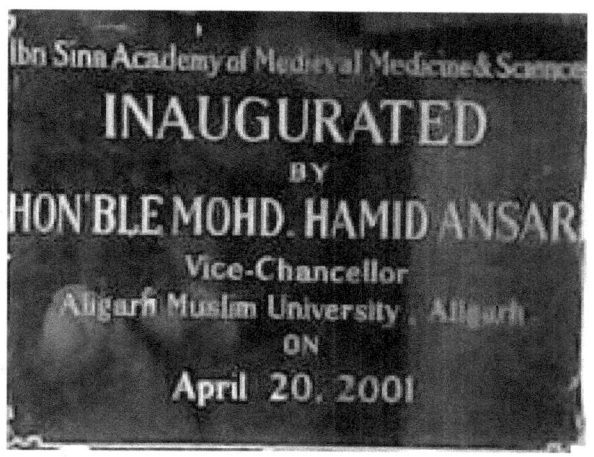

Foundation stone at the entrance gate of academy

under the aegis of **Tibbi Academy**. Majlis Ibn Sina was a sort of monthly discussion group. For instance, the first meeting of that Majlis was held to discuss typhoid.[5]

Tibbi Academy was itself formed in 1963 at Bhopal. In a note on page 4, of the first book of Tibbi Academy, on *Modern Times and Unani Medicine* the author Hakim Syed Zillur Rahman announced the establishment of Tibbi Academy with its clear objective: "to publicise the theoretical principles and practical ideas of Unani medicine, to publish the text of standard works of Unani medicine and also their translations... further, a learned and research oriented monthly journal".

From 1965 to 1970, a monthly journal with the title *Al-Hikmat* (in Urdu) from Delhi was published under the auspices of Tibbi Academy under the editorship of Syed Zillur Rahman Nadvi. The editor stated in the introduction of the first issue (May 1965, page 2) that the journal is being issued.

Further, besides the above-mentioned objectives, the editor

listed a couple of additional objectives, e.g., "the search of manuscripts of the Unani medicine, their edition and publication, ... to excite the feeling of the pressing need of Unani medicine literature, and to publish a standard book every year". He lamented that despite the publication of 30-40 Tibbi magazines in India, no learned journal of Unani medicine is being published. He stressed that *Al-Hikmat* would be a purely scholarly journal not confined to Unani medicine: It would include some articles on basic sciences, that is, zoology, botany, chemistry, physics, astronomy and philosophy.

In 1970, Hakim Syed Zillur Rahman renamed the Tibbi Academy as **Shifaul Mulk Memorial Committee** after his teacher, Shifaul Mulk Hakim Abdul Latif (29 April 1900–14 November 1970), former professor and principal of Ajmal Khan Tibbiya College, Aligarh Muslim University. The purpose of this memorial committee was the same as Tibbi Academy formed in 1963, except the widened scope of publications.

All these past establishments — **Tibbi Academy** (1963), **Majlis Ibn Sina** (1965) and **Shifaul Mulk Memorial Committee** (1970) — merged and came under one trustee organisation, i.e., **Ibn Sina Academy of Medieval Medicine and Sciences** in 2000. It was formally inaugurated on 21 April 2001.

2.5.3 Facilities

Hakim Zillur Rahman Library

The library houses one of the most precious and valuable collection of 20,000 printed books, 500 manuscripts,[6][7] some rare books, microfilms, compact discs and a large number of periodicals. Books in many languages like Arabic, Persian, Urdu, Sanskrit and English on subjects like History of Medicine and Sciences, Unani, Medieval medicine, Ilmul Advia (Pharmacology), Urdu Literature with special reference to Ghalib, Iqbal, Aligarh and Sir Syed Ahmad Khan, besides thousands of bound volumes of magazines are extant in this library.

The library is listed in the Directory of History of Medicine Collections, United States Department of Health and Human Services, National Library of Medicine, NIH.[8]

Hakim Karam Hussain Museum on History of Medicine and Sciences

Karam Husain Museum on History of Medicine and Sciences is an academic unit with collections and exhibitions. The main theme is the history of health and disease in a cultural perspective, with focus on the material and iconographic culture of medieval medicine and sciences. The museum has categorically the pictures and busts of physicians belonging to Mesopotamia, Babylonian, Egyptians, Greeks, Arab and Indian civilizations. In addition, medical manuscripts, catalogues, medical philately, medical souvenirs, memoirs of physicians including Nobel laureates, etc., are preserved and exhibited.

The museum is listed in the 'World's 10 weirdest medical museums', as per CNN Travel.[9]

Hakim Fazlur Rahman Museum on Arts, Culture and Orientalism

The museum has a large collection of coins, postage stamps, gemstones, paintings, engravings, watercolours, drawings, photographic print, utensils, garments including calico, busts, pens, memoirs and relics of some prominent personalities. In the museum, there are family collections like Prof. Syed Mahmood Husain Family Collection, Roohi Mabud Hasan Family Collection, etc.

Publication division under Shifaul Mulk Memorial Committee

The quarterly *Newsletter of Ibn Sina Academy* has had 52 issues published.[10] The academy has published a number of books on the history of medicine and sciences including pharmacology and literature.

Before the existence of Ibn Sina Academy, publications were done under the aegis of Tibbi Academy, formed in 1963. The first book of the Tibbi Academy was *Daur Jadeed aur Tibb* (Modern Times and Unani Medicine). From 1965 to 1970, a monthly Urdu journal, *Al-Hikmat*, was published under the auspices of Tibbi Academy. Under the Shifaul Mulk Memorial Committee many more publications came into existence and are known to the world of history of medicine. The Memorial Committee and Tibbi Academy are now a part of the Publication Division of Ibn Sina Academy.[11]

AIDS Cell

AIDS Cell of IAMMS was established in the year 2002 with Dr Imran Sabri as the founder Incharge of this prestigious institute. The Main AIM of the AIDS Cell is to spread awareness about AIDS in common population and newly graduated doctors. AIDS Cell of the academy is dedicated to improving lives, knowledge, and understanding worldwide through a highly diversified programme of research, education, and services in HIV/AIDS screening and prevention, care and treatment, reproductive health

and infectious diseases. AIDS Cell is a partner member of Global Health Council (USA) and the AIDS-Care-Watch Campaign (Thailand). It has a separate library of documents relevant to HIV/AIDS project management, research, and reproductive health issues apart from CD-ROMs, poster and books in several languages. AIDS Cell of IAMMS claims responsibility of holding Symposium on Medico-Social implication of the emerging epidemic of HIV/AIDS on India, Free Health check-up and Drug Distribution camp.

Ibn Sina Shifa Khana

For clinical studies of indigenous drugs, IAMMS is engaged in research and development in its clinical set-up, Ibn Sina Shifakhana, at Okhla Vihar, New Delhi.

Centre for Safety and Rational Use of Indian Systems of Medicine

The academy took a novel task of improving the use of Indian originated drugs and their adverse reaction monitoring under the establishment of Centre for Safety & Rational Use of Indian Systems of Medicine (CSRUISM) in 2005. CSRUISM receives many adverse drug reactions of herbs, which were never reported earlier. These reactions for their causal relationships are assessed according to Naranjo algorithm and WHO causality categories.

Ghalib Study Centre

This centre was set up to study Urdu poetry particularly of Mirza Ghalib. The centre has a largest collection on Ghalibiat (things related to Ghalib). It has many books and periodicals especially 'Ghalib Numbers' issued in different occasions, particularly on Ghalib's Centenary Celebration observed all over the world in 1969. In addition, there are hundreds of other poets' collection, memoirs and writings.

2.5.4 Annual events

- Ibn Sina Memorial Lecture: Courtesy, National Council for Promotion of Urdu Languages, Department of Education, Ministry of Human Resource Development, Government of India.

Series of Ibn Sina Memorial Lecture: - First Ibn Sina Memorial Lecture (2006) by Saiyid Hamid (Delhi) - Second Ibn Sina Memorial Lecture (2007) by Syed Mushirul Hasan (Delhi) - Third Ibn Sina Memorial Lecture (2008) by Syed Shahid Mehdi (Delhi) - Fourth Ibn Sina Memorial Lecture (2009) by Irfan Habib (Aligarh) - Fifth Ibn

Sina Memorial Lecture (2010) by Sadiqur Rahman Kidwai (Delhi) - Sixth Ibn Sina Memorial Lecture (2011) by Dr. Ahmad Abdul Hai (Patna) - Seventh Ibn Sina Memorial Lecture (2012) by Moosa Raza (Villupuram, Tamil Nadu) - Eight Ibn Sina Memorial Lecture (2013) by Muhammad Zakaria Virk (Ontario, Canada) - Ninth Ibn Sina Memorial Lecture (2015) by Dr. (Maulana) Kalbe Sadiq (Lucknow)

- Syed Shahid Mehdi delivering 3rd Ibn Sina Memorial Lecture

- Hakim Syed Zillur Rahman introducing Dr. S. Shahid Mehdi

- Prof. M. Nasim Ansari Memorial Lecture on World Health Day: Courtesy, SEARO, WHO, New Delhi.

Series of Prof. M. Nasim Ansari Memorial Lecture: - First Lecture (2007) by Dr. Md. Tauheed Ahmad (Aligarh) - Second Lecture (2008) by Dr. M. Habib Raza (Aligarh) - Third Lecture (2009) by Dr. D. P. Singh Toor (Delhi) - Fourth Lecture (2010) by Dr. Syed Badrul Hasan (Aligarh / Bhopal) - Fifth Lecture (2011) by Prof. M. Hanif Beg (Aligarh) - Sixth Lecture (2012) by Dr. Syed Badrul Hasan (Aligarh / Bhopal) - Seventh Lecture (2013) by Prof. Arshad Hafeez Khan (Aligarh) - Eighth Lecture (2014) by Prof. Saeeduzzafar Chaghtai (Aligarh) - Ninth Lecture (2015) by Prof. Mohd Zaheer (Aligarh)

- 2nd Prof. M. Nasim Ansari Memorial Lecture Delivered by Dr. M. Habib Raza

2.5.5   See also

- International Conference on "Life & Contribution of Ibn Sina"

- Collection of the Canon of Medicine (Al Qanoon fi al tibb by Ibn Sina)

- Galen's influence on Islamic medicine

- Kitab ila Aglooqan fi Shifa al Amraz

- 'Risalah al Nabidh' dated 1745AD

- Imad al-Din Mahmud ibn Mas'ud Shirazi

- Hakim Syed Karam Husain

- Hakim Syed Zillur Rahman (President)

- Mehdi Mohaghegh (Vice President)

- SM Razaullah Ansari (General Secretary)

- Syed Ziaur Rahman (Treasurer)

- Dawakhana Shifaul Amraz

2.5.6   References

[1] "Women's Health". International.

[2] "Essential Medicines". International.

[3] "CPTECH". International.

[4] "Climate Health". Health Prescriptions.

[5] Al-Hikmat, Issue of July 1965, Ed. Syed Zillur Rahman Nadvi, Tibbi Academy, Delhi,

[6] "Manuscripts Catalogues at Zillur Rahman Library". Microfilm Centre of India.

[7] "Manuscripts Libraries". Microfilm Centre of India.

[8] "Zillur Rahman Library". United States National Library of Medicine, National Institute of Health.

[9] "World's 10 weirdest medical museums". Bryan Pirolli for CNN, Travel (May 24, 2013).

[10] Newsletters of Ibn Sina Academy (NISA)

[11] Publication Division of Ibn Sina Academy

2.5.7   External links

- Photographs at Picaso Web Picture Gallery, Ibn Sina Academy

- Intute Resources, UK

- The Wellcome Trust Centre for the History of Medicine at UCL, UK

- Science Societies in India, IndianScience, India

- Acronym, IAMMS stands for Ibn Sina Academy of Medieval Medicine & Sciences

- In 2001 the agreement was signed with the Indian Ibn Sina Academy of Medieval Medicine and Sciences, Embassy of the Republic of Uzbekistan in Japan

- FaceBook

- AIDS Cell, IAMMS, MSMGF Secretariat, AIDS Project, LA, USA

- AIDS Cell News, Global Health Council, USA

- Releasing Ceremony of a Collection of Poem "Goonj", A.M.U. News And Views

- Prof Nasim Ansari Memorial Lecture on World Health Day, Indian Muslims News and Information

- Ek Shaam Mushtaq Yousufi Ke Naam, AMULIVE News

- Students receive AMU Alumni Association Michigan Scholarship, AMULIVE News

- WHD Events at Ibn Sina Academy, Aligarh, India, World Health Day 2010, World Health Organisation

- Exhibition and Painting Competition on SS Day

2.6 Jarrah (Surgeon)

Jarrah (Arabic: الجراح, Urdu: جراح) is an Arabic-language word for surgeon.

Whereas in Dekhani-Urdu the word *Jarrah* is termed for the Orthopaedists who are trained in the descipline of Unani medicine.[1]

In South India and particularly Hyderabad, India *Jarrah* are the bone setters, adjust joint dislocations and physiotherapists,[1] they use non-surgical means to treat fractures, dislocation, sports injuries and set the bone without applying any plaster. Jarrah do not rely on latest technology of treatment like X ray or any diagnosis and uses the art of treating orthopaedic problems with bare hands and supplementing it with regular essential oil massages and specially prepared Unani medicine pastes,[2] this is a long-term treatment, with minimum 3 weeks depending on the seriousness of case.

2.6.1 References

[1] "Hyderabad through the eyes of a voyager". timesofindia.indiatimes.com. 24 July 2011. Retrieved 4 September 2011.

[2] "Traditional bone setters unfazed by orthopaedists". thehansindia.info. September 4, 2011. Retrieved September 4, 2011.

2.6.2 External links

Traditional bone setters unfazed by orthopaedists

A bond with bones: hinduonnet.com

2.7 Lapidary (text)

A **lapidary** is a text, often a whole book, giving "information about the properties and virtues of precious and semi-precious stones", that is to say a work on gemology.[1] Lapidaries were very popular in the Middle Ages, when belief in the inherent power of gems for various purposes was widely held, and among the wealthy collecting jewels was often an

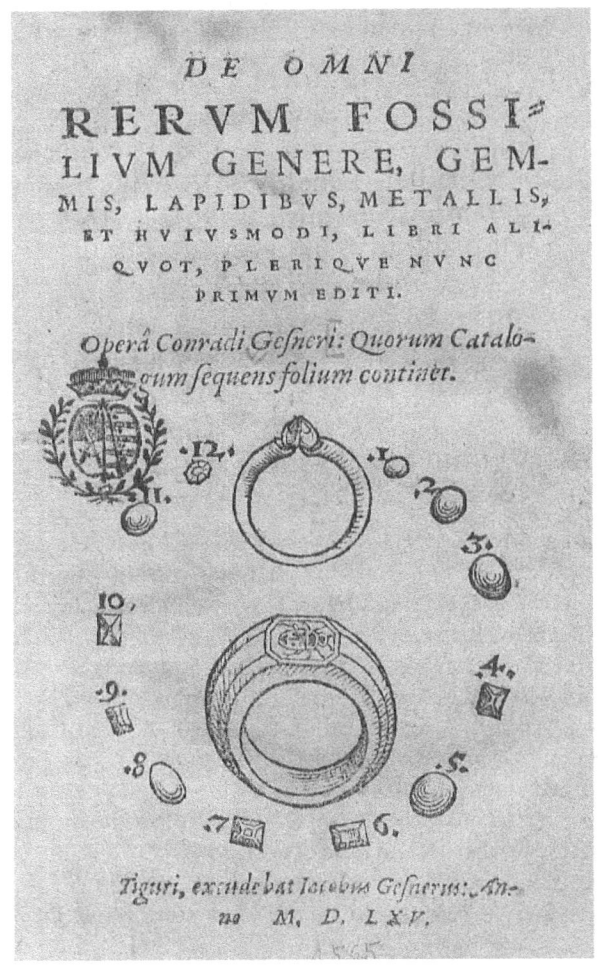

Title page of a printed lapidary by Conrad Gessner of 1565

obsession, as well as a popular way to store and transport capital.[2]

The medieval world had little systematic geological knowledge, and found it difficult to distinguish between many stones with similar colours, or the same stone found in a variety of colours.[3] Lapidaries are often found in conjunction with herbals, and as part of larger encyclopedic works. Belief in the powers of particular types of jewel to achieve effects such as protecting the wearer against diseases or other kinds of harm was strong in the Middle Ages, and explaining these formed much of the material in lapidaries. In the Middle Ages, scholars often distinguish "three different kinds of lapidaries: 1. the scientific lapidary 2. the magical or astrological lapidary and 3. the Christian symbolic lapidary", although contemporary readers would have regarded both the first two categories as representing scientific treatments.[4]

The objects regarded as "stones" in the classical, medieval Renaissance periods included many now classified as metallic compounds such as cinnabar, haemetite, calamine, or organic or fossil substances including pearl, coral, amber, and the mythical lyngurium described below.[5]

There were traditions of lapidary texts outside Europe, in the Islamic world as well as East Asia. The Chinese tradition was for long essentially concerned with the aesthetic qualities of stones, but by the later Middle Ages were influenced by the classical Western tradition, as transmitted through Islamic texts.[6]

2.7.1 Main sources

The tradition goes back to ancient Mesopotamia with books like Abnu šikinšu. Theophrastus (died c. 287 BC) treated rocks and other minerals as well as gems, and remained a significant indirect source for the scientific tradition; he was all but unknown in Europe in the Middle Ages, and not translated into Latin until the 15th century.[7] He attempted to fill out with specifics the general remarks on minerals of Aristotle, and took an approach more compatible with modern concepts of mineralogy than any other writer of a full-length treatise on the subject until Georgius Agricola in the 16th century, widely recognised as the "father" of modern mineralogy. Both concentrated on the appearance of a wide range of minerals, where they came from, and how they were extracted and used.[8] While Pliny and others wrote on how to detect fake or imitation gems, some, like Jean d'Outremeuse (d. 1400), described how to make them in coloured glass, which by the Late Middle Ages was recommended for use in church metalwork.[9]

Most classical lapidaries are lost; of the 38 works listed by Pliny (in Book XXXVII), only Theophrastus' text survives.[10] There are hundreds of different medieval texts, but most are mainly based on a number of large works which were redacted, translated and adapted in various ways to suit the needs of the individual manuscript. The oldest of these sources was Pliny the Elder's *Natural History* from the 1st century AD, Book 37 of which covered gems, drawing on Theophrastus and other classical predecessors. Solinus was another ancient source, and Isidore of Seville an early medieval one. Later works, which also drew on Arabic sources (Avicenna's work was available in Latin), included the verse *De Gemmis* (or *De Lapidibus*) by Bishop Marbode of Rennes (d. 1123), the most popular late medieval lapidary, describing 60 stones, and works by Arnold of Saxony, Vincent of Beauvais and that traditionally attributed (probably wrongly) to Albertus Magnus.[11] Versions of Marbode's work were translated into eight languages, including Hebrew and Irish, and 33 manuscripts survive of the English version alone.[12]

As in other areas, medieval scholarship was highly conservative. Theophrastus had described lyngurium, a gemstone supposedly formed of the solidified urine of the lynx (the best ones coming from wild males), which was included in "almost every medieval lapidary" until it gradually disappeared from view in the 17th century.[13]

2.7.2 Medicine

Just as drugs derived from plants were and are important in medicine, it seemed natural to the ancient and medieval mind that minerals also had medical properties (and indeed many mineral-derived chemicals are still in medical use). Saint Thomas Aquinas, the dominant theologian of the Late Middle Ages, propounded the view that the whole of the natural world had ultimately been created by God for the benefit of man, leading medieval Christians to expect to find beneficial uses for all materials.[14] Lapidaries listed the medical benefits of particular gems, with "the most common method of medical application" being wearing the stone on one's person in a jewellery setting, for example in a ring. Open-backed settings allowing direct contact between the skin and stone were encouraged; otherwise the stone might simply be held against the skin.[15] Other forms of application included ointments containing ground stones or taking the stone internally in ground form, often as part of a cocktail of several different herbal, mineral and other ingredients; this seems to have become especially often mentioned in the 16th and 17th centuries.[16] There were other methods of application; Theophrastus is much less concerned with medical aspects of his subject than the writers of later lapidaries, but he notes that smaragus is good for the eyes, and operates by being looked at.[17]

Stones were covered in other general medical books, ranging from the 1st century Greek *De Materia Medica* by Dioscurides to a wide range of Early Modern medical self-help books.[18]

2.7.3 Christian symbolism

A school of lapidaries expounded the symbolism of gems mentioned in the Bible, especially two sets of precious and semi-precious stones listed there. The first of these were the twelve jewels, in engraved gem form, on the Priestly breastplate described in the Book of Exodus (Exodus 28:15–19), and the second the twelve stones mentioned in the Book of Revelation as forming the foundation stones of the New Jerusalem (Revelation 21:18–20)—eight of these are the same (or were in the Vulgate translation). The late Anglo-Saxon Old English Lapidary took the latter group as its subject. The symbolism of these sets had been explored by theologians since Saints Jerome and Augustine.[19] Various other schemes were developed, linking stones to particular saints, classes of angels, and other areas of Christianity.[20]

2.7.4 Astrology

Another type of lapidary dealt with the astrological relationships and significance of gems; one of the largest was the *Lapidary of Alfonso X* or "Alfonso the Learned", King of Castile (r. 1252–1284), which was compiled for him by other authors, mostly Muslim. This was in several parts and set out the relationships between the Signs of the Zodiac, with each degree of each sign relating to a stone, and the astrological planets and other bodies, again related to particular stones. The strength of the medical and magical properties of stones was said to vary with the movements of the heavenly bodies that controlled them. [21]

2.7.5 Notes

[1] Glick et al, 306; Vauchez, 821

[2] Wheaton

[3] Harris, 15–17

[4] Wheaton, quoted; Harris, 11 note 15, 35–39. Harris, 11–15 gives her own classification into six types.

[5] Harris, 14–16, 48–49

[6] Harris, 21–22

[7] Walton, 359–360; Wheaton

[8] Harris, 45–50

[9] Vauchez, 822; Harris, 17

[10] Harris, 55

[11] Glick et al, 306; Vauchez, 821–822; Harris, 19–20

[12] Walton, 362

[13] Walton, 365, quoted

[14] Harris, 1–2, 41–42, 45

[15] Harris, 8–9, 8 quoted

[16] Harris, 9–10

[17] Harris, 49

[18] Harris, 50–55, 13–14, 30–34, 42–44

[19] Vauchez, 821; Walton, 362

[20] Wheaton

[21] Evans, 424–426; Nunemaker, 103

2.7.6 References

- Cherry, John, *Medieval Goldsmiths*, The British Museum Press, 2011 (2nd edn.), ISBN 9780714128238

- Evans, Joan, "The 'Lapidary' of Alfonso the Learned", *The Modern Language Review*, Vol. 14, No. 4 (Oct., 1919), pp. 424–426, Modern Humanities Research Association, JSTOR

- Glick, Thomas F., Livesey, Steven John, Wallis, Faith, eds., "Lapidary" in *Medieval Science, Technology And Medicine: An Encyclopedia*, Volume 11 of The Routledge encyclopedias of the Middle Ages, 2005, Routledge, ISBN 0415969301, 9780415969307, google books

- Harris, Nichola Erin, *The idea of lapidary medicine*, 2009, Rutgers University, Ph.D. dissertation (book forthcoming), available online as PDF

- Nunemaker, J. Horace, "The Madrid Manuscript of the Alfonsine Lapidaries", *Modern Philology*, Vol. 29, No. 1 (Aug., 1931), pp. 101–104, University of Chicago Press, JSTOR

- Thorndike, Lynn, "Some Unpublished Minor Works Bordering on Science Written in the Late Fifteenth Century", *Speculum*, Vol. 39, No. 1 (Jan., 1964), pp. 85–95, Medieval Academy of America, JSTOR

- Vauchez, André, Lapidge, Michael (eds), *Encyclopedia of the Middle Ages: A-J*, Volume 1 of *Encyclopedia of the Middle Ages*, 2000, Routledge, ISBN 1579582826, 9781579582821, google books

- Walton, S.A., *Theophrastus on Lyngurium: medieval and early modern lore from the classical lapidary tradition*, 2001, *Annals of Science*, 2001 Oct;58(4):357-79, PDF on Academia.edu

- "Wheaton": "Medieval Lit Bibliography – Stones", Wheaton College, Illinois

2.7.7 Further reading

- Evans, Joan, *Magical Jewels of the Middle Ages and the Renaissance, Particularly in England*, 1922, Oxford (often reprinted)

- Riddle, John M., *Marbode of Rennes' De lapidibus: considered as a medical treatise*, 1977, Wiesbaden

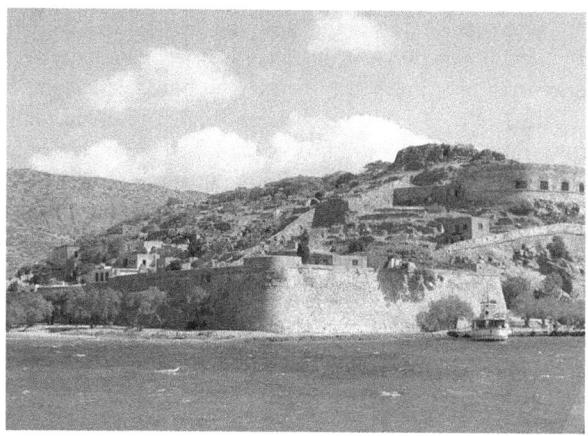

Spinalonga on Crete, Greece, one of the last leper colonies in Europe, closed in 1957.

2.8   Leper colony

A **leper colony**, **leprosarium**, or **lazar house** is a place to quarantine people with leprosy (Hansen's disease). The term *lazaretto* can refer to quarantine sites, which were at some time also leper colonies.

2.8.1   History

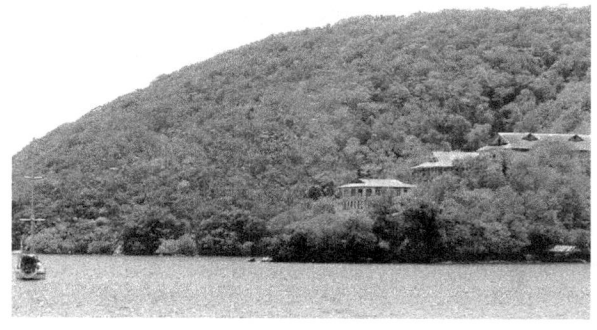

Abandoned nun's quarters at the leper colony on Chacachacare Island in Trinidad and Tobago.

Leper colonies or houses became widespread in the Middle Ages, particularly in Europe and India, and often run by monastic orders. Historically, leprosy has been greatly feared because it causes visible disfigurement and disability, was incurable, and was commonly believed to be highly contagious. A leper colony administered by a Roman Catholic order was often called a lazar house, after Lazarus, the patron saint of lepers.[1]

Some colonies were located on mountains or in remote locations in order to ensure quarantine, some on main roads, where donations would be made for their upkeep. Debate exists over the conditions found within historical leper colonies; while they are currently thought to have been grim and neglected places, there are some indications that life within a leper colony or house was no worse than the life of other, non-quarantined individuals. There is even doubt that the current definition of leprosy can be retrospectively applied to the Medieval condition. What was classified as leprosy then covers a wide range of skin conditions that would be classified as distinct afflictions today.[2]

Some leper colonies issued their own money (such as tokens), in the belief that allowing lepers to handle regular money could spread the disease.[3][4]

The last existing leper colony in Europe is Tichileşti in Romania.

2.8.2   Political aspects

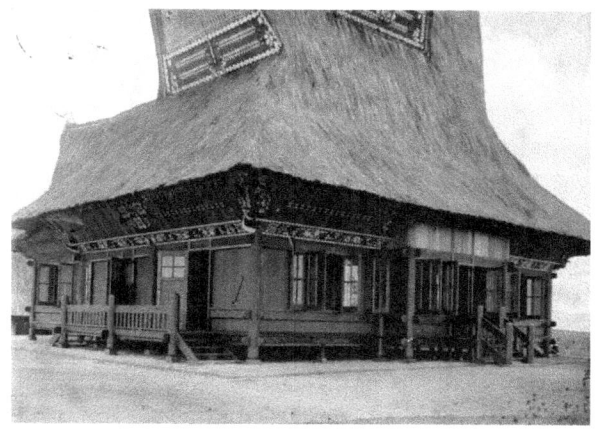

Laoe Si Momo (Spring Water) leper colony founded on August 25, 1906 in the Batak region of Sumatra, 10 kilometers from Kaban Jahe. Within five months it was home to 72 lepers and by April 1921 colony included 280. The patients lived in small houses

In 2001, government-run leper colonies in Japan came under judicial scrutiny, leading to the determination that the Japanese government had mistreated the patients, and the district court ordered Japan to pay compensation to former patients.[5] In 2002, a formal inquiry into these colonies was set up, and in March 2005, the policy was strongly denounced. "Japan's policy of absolute quarantine... did not have any scientific grounds."[6] The inquiry denounced not only the government and the doctors who were involved with the policy, but also the court that repeatedly ruled in favor of the government when the policy was challenged, as well as the media, which failed to report the plight of the victims.

2.8.3 See also

- History of leprosy

- Kalawao County, Hawaii

- Leprosy colony money

2.8.4 References

[1] "Patron Saints Index: Saint Lazarus".

[2] Archived October 23, 2008 at the Wayback Machine

[3] Unique experiment with currency notes(1970) Isaac Teoh, The Star, January–February, p7.

[4] The numismatic aspects of leprosy(1993), McFadden, RR, Grost J, Marr DF. p.21 D.C.McDonald Associates, Inc. U.S.A.

[5] "Koizumi apologises for leper colonies". *BBC News*. 2001-05-25. Retrieved 2007-03-20.

[6] "Japan's leprosy policy denounced". *BBC News*. 2005-03-02. Retrieved 2007-03-20.

2.9 MacDunleavy/MacNulty physicians of Tirconnell

The **MacDunleavy/MacNulty physicians of Tirconnell** (sometimes also noted to include the MacKinley)[1] were originally of one of Gaelic Ireland's royal families, which was, also, one of its ancient hereditary medical families. In the mid to late middle ages, likely, because of, their, unique status as then former royals and their Latin schooling, Tirconnell's MacDonlevy/MacNulty physicians provided an important conduit of communication between Ireland's (really the Celtic Nations) and the rest of Western Europe's medical communities.

The reputation, skill and influence of Tirconnell's MacDonlevy/MacNulty physicians survives, even, into modern times. Dr. Sir Arthur MacNalty (variant of MacNulty),[2] whose father was the physician F.C. MacNalty, M.D., carried on this tradition, becoming, eventually, the 8th Chief Medical Officer, a physician renowned in several medical specialties in his lifetime,[3] an acquaintance of Sir Winston Churchill[4] and the top British government health official during his administration, and is, to today, renowned as a historian (particularly, of published medieval medical history reconstructions).[5] A ground breaking medical scientist, MacNalty was the first to use electrocardiography in clinical medicine. In 1908, Arthur MacNalty and Thomas Lewis (cardiologist) teamed to employ electrocardiography to diagnose Heart block.[6] Based largely on his for

then advanced understandings of the relation between endocrine function and neurological disorders and the relation between human immune function and human nutrition, in the late 1930s, Sir Arthur became the first national public health official known to have warned of the dangers of indiscriminant use of Anti-obesity medications (or what was then known as "dosing") and against fad diet (or what was then known as "slimming").[7][8]

2.9.1 Renown of Irish physicians during the middle ages

Through medieval times, most Irish physicians were educated domestically under a hereditary apprenticeship system. In the middle ages, likely, because of this warehousing of over a millennium of empirically accumulated knowledge of medicaments and battlefield surgery techniques, Irish physicians and surgeons were renowned throughout the western world. An Irish king's personal surgeon accompanied him to battle, and many an Irish king owed his life manifold times over to the skills of his surgeon. More than a thousand years before the Frenchman René Laennec in 1816 reinvented or expropriated from the Irish the stethoscope and the Scotsman Joseph Lister, 1st Baron Lister introduced acid poultices for sanitation of healing surgical wounds, Irish physicians employed elk horns of the same general hollowed conical configuration as early stethoscopes and for the same exact purpose of during auscultation amplifying the sound of the body's cardiac pulse and fire cupping therapy (the vestiges of which can be observed to this day in traditional Chinese medicine practice) to drain the purulence from healing wounds, while also sanitising them by heating of local atmosphere and tissue.[9][10]

2.9.2 Emigration to "Tir Chonaill" or land of The O'Donnell

Upon the late 12th century collapse of the ancient eastern Irish Kingdom of Ulidia, it is reputed that many of the kingdom's ruling MacDunleavy/MacNulty, who, again, were also one of the ancient hereditary medical families of Ireland, sought political asylum in the western Irish Kingdom of Tirconnell,[11] the last standing Gaelic sovereignty, which boundaries were contemporaneous with those of modern County Donegal, where they were named to the high Gaelic status of "ollamh leighis" or the official physicians to the O'Donnells dynasty kings of Tyrconnell (E., var. spell., "Tyrconnell", I. "Tir Chonaill", abbr. "Tir") and to a historical certainty there adopted the agnomen I. Ultach (var. I. spell. Ultagh or Ultaigh, L. Ulidian), which as earlier notated is said to have evolved by prefixing of the Gaelic language element "Mac" to the element Ultagh to form the

Irish "patronymic" surname Mac an Ultaigh (English Mac-Nulty or McNulty).[12][13][14]

2.9.3 Communication with medical fraternities on the European continent

Unlike most of Ireland's other physicians, many of the Mac-Donlevy/MacNulty physicians of Tirconnell were also educated by medical faculty at Universities on the European continent at a time when continental European medicine was despite the work of Andreas Vesalius and other medical empiricists still mired in the philosophical musings of Galen and other medical rationalists. Tir Chonaill's Mac-Dunleavy/MacNulty physicians provided an important conduit between continental Europe's and Ireland's philosophically divergent medical communities. They maintained discourse with the great continental European medical schools of the time, including at Toulouse, Louvain (Leuven), Paris, Montpellier, Bologna and Padua. Ireland's MacDonleavy/MacNulty physicians both introduced to Ireland continental European medical scholarship and to the European continent Irish medical empiricism, which foreshadowed, if it did not, itself, actually anticipate, the later broader introduction of scientific method to western medicine and surgery by surgeons like the Frenchman Ambroise Paré and Scotsman John Hunter.

2.9.4 List of Tir Chonaill's MacDonlevy/McNulty "ollahm leighis"

This is a partial list, based on the incomplete record of the Annals of the Four Masters or the Irish Annals, of members of the MacDonlevy/McNulty family, who in the Kingdom of Tir Chonaill were official physicians to its O'Donnell dynasty kings.[15]

- Muiris MacDonlevy (d. 1395) is the first member of the MacDonlevy/McNulty family actually entered in the Irish Annals as an I. "ollah lieghis chenel Conaill" or official physician to the O'Donnell dynasty.

- By his agnomens Paul Ultach or Paul the Ulidian, Muiris's father is also mentioned at this 1395 A.D. entry to be an "ollahm lieghis", who flourished both before and after Muiris.

- Murtough Ultaigh Donlevy is recorded as having been an "ollav" or the official physician to the O'Donnell dynasty in Tir Chonaill in the year (ol. 1497).[16]

- Donnchadh mac Eoghan Ó Duinnshléibhe, Donnchadh MacDonlevy, M.D. or Donough Ultach or Dunlevy (d. 1526 or 1528) is entered as an "ollahm leighis"

and as the son of an Eoghan, who was prior an "ollahm lieghis." Donnchadh was educated on the continent at Paris.[17] He was famed for his general learning and, too, his great wealth.

- Donnell Ultaigh Donlevy (d. 1567), the son of a, then, but unnamed Ultaigh "ollav" to the O'Donnell in Tir Chonaill, is recorded as having been slain in the year 1567.

- Eoghan MacDonlevy, M.D. or Owen Ultach (d. 1586) was the son of Donnchadh and, also, educated at Paris. Likewise known for his general learning, this "ollahm leighis" was further considered throughout Ireland and much of Europe as the finest physician of his time. His skills are not only recounted by the Irish Annals and at the Dictionary of National Biography but also by Stanihurst.

The Annals note further that the branch of the MacDonlevy, who had been the official physicians to the O'Donnell dynasty kings of Tir Chonaill, still existed near Kilmacrenan, County Donegal in the early 17th century.

2.9.5 Example Cormac MacDonlevy

Cormac MacDonlevy (E. var. MacDunleavy, anglicised from I. Mac or Ó Duinnshléibhe) (Ultach) (fl. c. 1460) was an influential medieval Irish physician and medical scholar. He is famed for advancing Irish medieval medical practice by, for the first time, translating seminal continental European medical texts from Latin to vernacular. His translations provided the, then, exclusively, Gaelic language speaking majority of Irish physicians with their first reference access to these texts.

In or about 1470, Cormac MacDonlevy, M.B.[18] commenced the daunting 12-year task of first translating the French physician Bernard of Gordon's most celebrated and extensive medical work, the *Lilium medicine*[19] (1320), from Latin to Irish.[20] Thereafter, as it had some 150 years earlier with the continental European medical community, the monumental *Lilium medicine* or English "Lily of Medicine" achieved great popularity among the medical community of the Celtic nations. Cormac, also, first translated Gordon's *De pronosticis*[21] (c. 1295) and Gaulteris Agilon's *De dosibus*[22] (c. 1250) from Latin into Irish. Gaulteris' *De dosibus* is a pharmaceutical tract and well utilised historical source, providing a concise introduction to the basic principles and operations of medieval European pharmacy. Cormac, too, first translated from Latin to Irish the French surgeon Gui de Chuliac's *Chirurgia*[23] (c. 1363) and, also, 5 other major Continental European medical texts in addition to those hereto cited.[24]

2.9.6 Example Nellanus Glacanus

Tradition is that the MacDonlevy/MacNulty physicians educated in the medical arts L. Nellanus Glacanus, originally, Niall Ó Glacáin of Tir Chonaill or Donegal, and it is quite probable that they would have provided this Tir Chonaill native his medical education. After his reputed education and training under the MacDonleavy/McNulty, and, anyway, in the modern area of County Donegal, Republic of Ireland, Glacanus became a famed physician, professor of medicine and medical researcher on the continent. He was physician to Louis XIII of France and may have attended Aodh Ruadh Ó Domhnaill in 1602 at his deathbed at Simancas Castle in Spain. Glacanus was a professor and researcher at the University of Bologna. Glacanus applied empirical method to pioneer the field of forensic anatomy and pathology. His autopsies first described the petechial haemorrhages of the lung and swelling of the spleen incident of bubonic plague (*Tractatus de Peste*, 1629), and he early elucidated on the empirical method of differential diagnosis to the continental European medical community (*Cursus Medicus*, 1655).[25]

2.9.7 References

[1] Rev. Patrick Woulfe, Priest of the Diocese of Limerick, Member of the Council, National Academy of Ireland, *Irish Names and Surnames*, 1967 Baltimore: Genealogical Publishing Company, in Irish and English, pp. 319 and 355–356 – One scholarly contention is that both the surnames MacNulty (from I. Mac "son" an "of" or "an" Ultaigh or, var., Ultach L. "Ulidian") and MacKinley (from I. Mac "son" an "of" or "an" Léigh (liaig) (liaig) "leech" for "physician") originated during the middle ages in western Ireland's Kingdom of Tirconnell. Scholars, so contending, equate the McKinley, the McNulty and the Dunleavy.

[2] Elsdon C. Smith , *New Dictionary of American Family Names*, New York Harper & Row 1956, 1973, pp 330, 366, 387, 375

[3] Sir Weldon Dalrymple-Champneys, Royal College of Physicians, Lives of Fellows, Munk's Roll, Vol. VI (1966–1975), p. 321

[4] *Winston Spencer Churchill, Servant of Crown and Commonwealth. A Tribute By Various Hands presented to Him on His Eightieth Birthday* (1954, London, Cassell & Company), Sir James Marchant (Ed.), contributors of impressions from personal acquaintance include Sir Arthur Salusbury MacNalty

[5] , *Encyclopedia Britannica Online*, Henry VIII, ARTICLE, Additional Reading, "Arthur Salusbury MacNalty, *Henry VIII: The Difficult Patient* (1952), remains the best introduction to the medical history (which had important political consequences)."

[6] "A note on the simultaneous occurrence of sinus and ventricular rhythm in man", Lewis T, Macnalty AS, J Physiol. 1908 Dec 15;37(5–6):445-58

[7] , Launceston, Tasmania, Australia, *Examiner*, Friday, 21 January 1938, p 14, which states in postscript "However, the sex which for many years injured its health by tight lacing is not likely to be deterred from slimming by such considerations, The dictates of fashion will be paramount." Sir Arthur was particularly concerned with the neurological side effects of the then popular practice of dosing with thyroid extract to lose weight and, also, use of the then much vaunted weight loss drug dinitrophenol, which his report found killed as many patients as it reduced in girth, as well as, the compromise of the malnourished's immune system and their consequent, often, inability to resist infectious diseases like the then endemic tuberculosis (archaic "epidemics of consumption").

[8] See, also, , *Sidney Morning Herald*, 17 Nov 1937, p 10.

[9] P.W. Joyce *A Social History of Ancient Ireland* London: Longmans, Green & Co. (1903) Vol. 1 Chapter 18 "Medicine and Medical Doctors" pp 597–631

[10] See entirety of both A. Nic Donnchadha, "Medical Writing in Irish", in *2000 Years of Irish Medicine*, J.B. Lyons, ed., Dublin, Eirinn Health Care Publications © 2000 (Nic Donchadha contribution reprinted from *Irish Journal of Medicine*, Vol. 169, No. 3, pp 217–220) and Susan Wilkinson, "Early Medical Education in Ireland", *Irish Migration Studies in Latin America*, Vol. 6, No. 3 (November 2008). Both of the preceding articles also discuss the high status that physicians were accorded in Gaelic society. Wilkinson at page 158 specifically discusses the particularly high status of "ollahm leighis".

[11] *The Oxford Companion to Irish History*, 2nd ed., S.J. Connolly, ed., Oxford: Oxford University Press © 1998, 2002, ISBN 0-19-866270-X, pp. 350–351

[12] Edward MacLysaght, *The Surnames of Ireland*, 5th Edition, Irish Academic Press, Dublin, 1980, p 238, 292, who cites to 2 entries in The Annals of the Four Masters, which is a historical chronicle that records, among other matter, the births and deaths of Gaelic nobility. The first entry cited is an entry recording the 1395 A.D. death of a Maurice, the son of one "Paul Utach", who is, himself, recorded there to be "Chief Physician of Tyrconnell" and also as "Paul the Ulidian". It is there in the *Annals* further stated by its authors of the father Paul Ultach that "This is the present usual Irish name of the Mac Donlevy, who were originally chiefs of Ulidia. The branch of the family who became physicians to O'Donnell are still extant (at time of compilation of the Annals in the 17th century just after the fall of the last Gaelic sovereignty of Tyrconnell in 1607), near Kilmacrenan, in the county of Donegal." The second citation is to an entry recording the 1586 A.D. death of "Owen Utach", who is therein noted to be a particularly distinguished and skilled physician. The *Annal* 's compilers further elaborate of Owen Ultach at this

entry that "His real name was Donlevy or, Mac Donlevy. He was physician to O'Donnell (Aodh Ruadh Ó Domhnaill)."

[13] Other prominent MacDunleavy/MacNulty physicians of Gaelic Ireland's Tirconnell noted in *The Annals of the Four Masters* include a 1527 entry for Donnchadh mac Eoghan Ó Duinnshléibhe

[14] Rev. Patrick Woulfe, Priest of the Diocese of Limerick, Member of the Council, National Academy of Ireland, *Irish Names and Surnames*, 1967 Baltimore: Genealogical Publishing Company, in Irish and English, p.356

[15] Dictionary of National Biography, ibid, p. 52 and the Irish Annals are the basic sources for this Article section. Sources at particular entries supplement as to the specific additional statements there referenced.

[16] G.H. Hack Genealogical History of the Donlevy Family Columbus, Ohio: printed for private distribution by Chaucer Press, Evans Printing Co. (1901), pp 18, 21 (Wisconsin Historical Society Copy), also, at same pages source for Donnell Ultaigh Donlevy, further down on list of Articles main text

[17] A New History of Modern Ireland (Early modern Ireland 1534–1691) T. Moody, F. Mortin, F. Byrned, eds., NY: Oxford University Press © 1987, 1993 p 611

[18] The degree is noted in British Library MS 333, fol. 113v25, which manuscript copy of the Irish *De dosibus* was later scribed than the Royal Irish Academy copy of the same appearing in reference below. The British Library copy is dated 1459, so Cormac must have completed this work of translation and his formal medical education sometime earlier than that date. It is unknown where Cormac obtained his medical degree, but it was, likely, from a Continental European university, as, again, institutionalized medical training in Ireland at the time was by apprenticeship, really, pupilage, with medical knowledge, generally, being passed from physician father to student son.

[19] Dublin Royal Irish Academy, MS 443 (24 p 14), pp 1–327, undated (Cormac's translation of this work, though, was completed by 1482, which is the date appearing on a later scribed copy of the Irish *Lilium*, which copy is housed as Egerton MS 89, fols. 13ra1-192vb13 at the British Library.)

[20] See French Wikipedia article Bernard de Gordon. See, also, A. Nic Donnchadha, ibid, at page 218 at paragraphs 5, 6 and 7 under the subtitle "Medical texts in Irish".

[21] Dublin Royal Irish Academy, MS 439 (3C19), fols. 241–288, undated (The translation of the *De pronosticis* was also digested in 1468 as National Library of Ireland, MS G11, pp 425–38 and, so was completed by Cormac prior to this date.)

[22] British Library Harley MS 546, fols. 1r-11r (This translation has also been republished modernly as Shawn Sheehan, *An Irish Version of Gaulterus (sic) "De dosibus"*, Washington, D.C., Catholic University of America 1938 and with

Cormac's Irish translation and an English translation set side by side on adjoining of its 185 pages.)

[23] National Library of Ireland, MSG 453, fols. 110-27, undated (The translation of the work was also digested with date 1514 as British Library Arundel MS 333, fol. 37va17-21, fol. 35v20-29, and, so, Cormac had completed it at least by such date.)

[24] A. Nic Donnchadha, ibid, at page 218 at paragraphs 5, 6 and 7 under the subtitle "Medical texts in Irish".

[25] David Murphy "Niall O'Glacan" *Dictionary of Irish Biography ... to the year 2002*, James McGuire and James Quinn, eds., Cambridge, 2009.

2.10 Matthaeus Silvaticus

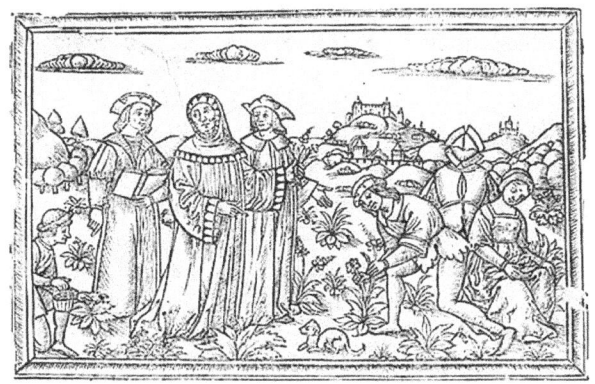

Matthaeus Silvaticus teaching his students about medicinal plants in his physic garden in Salerno, from the frontispiece to a 1526 edition of Opus Pandectarum Medicinae

Matthaeus Silvaticus or **Mattheus Sylvaticus** (c. 1280 – c. 1342) was a medieval Latin medical writer and botanist. His notability is for a 650-page encyclopedia about medicating agents (a pharmacopoeia) which he completed about year 1317 under the Latin title *Pandectarum Medicinae* or *Pandectae Medicinae* (English: *Encyclopedia of Medicines*). Most of the medicating agents were botanicals ("herbal medicines"). The presentation is in alphabetical order. The bulk of what he says is compiled from earlier medicine books, including books by Dioscorides, Avicenna, Serapion the Younger, and Simon of Genoa.[1] As an indication of its popularity in late medieval Europe, the *Pandectarum Medicinae* was printed in at least eleven editions in various countries between the invention of the printing press and 1500.[2]

Mattheus Silvaticus was born in northern Italy, probably Mantua.[3] He was a student and teacher in botany and medicine at the School of Salerno in southern Italy.

The medical school in Salerno was influenced by Arabic-to-Latin translations of Arabic medical literature. As one indication of Arabic influence, 233 of 487 plant names that Matthaeus used were Latinizations of Arabic plant names.[4] Many of those Latinized Arabic names had little circulation in Latin. Native Latin names existed for some of them, in which case Matthaeus also presents the native Latin name as well. In some cases he prefers to give primary status to the Arabic name in preference to the classical Latin name. In other cases he gives primary status to the Latin name and just mentions what the Arabic name is.

The *Pandectarum Medicinae* is an encyclopedia with almost no original thinking. It has considerable value to historians as a document reflecting the state of pharmacology and medicine in Europe in the late medieval era. The method of presentation in *Pandectarum Medicinae* is that a medicinal substance is named together with very brief identifying information and then follows several lengthier summaries or quotations from several well-known medical authorities about the substance's properties and uses. The medical authorities are either (A) the particular ancient Greek medical writers that were widely read by the medieval Arabs (particularly Diosorides and Galen) or else (B) Arabic medical writers (particularly Serapion the Younger and Avicenna).

Part of Matthaeus's encyclopedia was taken from a shorter work by Simon of Genoa (aka Simon Januensis) entitled *Synonyma Medicinae*, which was written a few decades earlier and which is a dictionary of medicines rather than an encyclopedia.[5]

2.10.1 References

[1] "The Encyclopedia of Medicaments - Pandectarum Medicinae". *World Digital Library*. May 11, 2013. Retrieved 2014-03-01.

[2] *Pandectarum Medicinae* at http://www.interzone.com/~{}cheung/SUM.dir/med43.html. A number of 15th century editions of the *Pandectarum* are online at Digitale-Sammlungen.de.

[3] *Dictionnaire historique de la médecine ancienne et moderne*, by N.F.J. Eloy (year 1778).

[4] Matteo Silvatico @ SummaGallicana.it (in Italian language).

[5] A late-15th-century edition of Simon of Genoa's *Synonyma Medicinae* is online at Google Books (in Latin). A 19th-century publication of a 15th-century Latin medical botany dictionary called the *Alphita* contains, in its 19th-century footnotes, many cross-references to Mattheus Silvaticus and Simon Januensis. It is downloadable at *Alphita*.

2.10.2 External links

- A short biography of Mattheus Silvaticus together with a description of his *Pandectarum Medicinae* is at SummaGallicana.it (in Italian language)

- Different editions of the *Opus Pandectarum* (aka *Liber Pandectae*) as printed in Latin in the late 15th century are online at Digitale-Sammlungen.de (year 1498), Digitale-Sammlungen.de (year 1488), Gallica.BNF.fr (year 1480).

2.11 Plague doctor

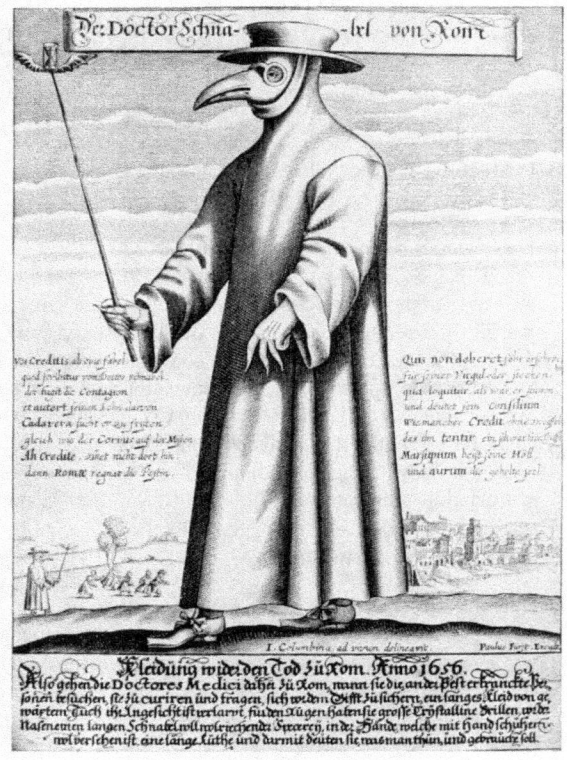

Doktor Schnabel von Rom ("Doctor Beak of Rome" in German) with a satirical Latin/German macaronic poem ('Vos Creditis, als eine Fabel, / quod scribitur vom Doctor Schnabel') in octosyllabic rhyming couplets. Engraving by Paul Fürst, 1656.

A **plague doctor** was a special medical physician who treated those who had the plague.[1] They were specifically hired by towns that had many plague victims in times of epidemics. Since the city was paying their salary, they treated everyone: both the rich and the poor.[2] However, some plague doctors were known for charging patients and their families extra for special treatments and/or false cures.[3] They were not normally profession-ally trained experienced physicians or surgeons, and often were second-rate doctors unable to otherwise run a success-ful medical business or young physicians trying to establish themselves.[1]

Plague doctors by their covenant treated plague patients and were known as municipal or "community plague doctors", whereas "general practitioners" were separate doctors and both might be in the same European city or town at the same time.[1][4][5][6] In France and the Netherlands plague doc-tors often lacked medical training and were referred to as "empirics". In one case a plague doctor had been a fruit salesman before his employment as a physician.[7]

In the seventeenth and eighteenth centuries, some doctors wore a beak-like mask which was filled with aromatic items. The masks were designed to protect them from putrid air, which (according to the miasmatic theory of disease) was seen as the cause of infection. Thus:

> The nose half a foot long, shaped like a beak, filled with perfume with only two holes, one on each side near the nostrils, but that can suffice to breathe and to carry along with the air one breathes the impression of the drugs enclosed further along in the beak. Under the coat we wear boots made in Moroccan leather (goat leather) from the front of the breeches in smooth skin that are attached to said boots and a short-sleeved blouse in smooth skin, the bottom of which is tucked into the breeches. The hat and gloves are also made of the same skin ... with spectacles over the eyes.
> — [8]

2.11.1 History

The first epidemic of bubonic plague dates back to the mid 6th century, known as the Plague of Justinian.[9] The largest epidemic was the Black Death of Europe in the 14th cen-tury. In medieval times the large loss of people due to the bubonic plague in a town created an economic disaster. Community plague doctors were quite valuable and were given special privileges. For example, plague doctors were freely allowed to perform autopsies, which were otherwise generally forbidden in Medieval Europe, to research a cure for the plague.

In some cases, plague doctors were so valuable that when Barcelona dispatched two to Tortosa in 1650, outlaws cap-tured them *en route* and demanded a ransom. The city of Barcelona paid for their release.[5] The city of Orvieto hired Matteo fu Angelo in 1348 for 4 times the normal rate of a

doctor of 50-florin per year.[5] Pope Clement VI hired sev-eral extra plague doctors during the Black Death plague. They were to attend to the sick people of Avignon. Of eigh-teen doctors in Venice, only one was left by 1348: five had died of the plague, and twelve were missing and may have fled.[10]

2.11.2 Costume

Main article: Plague doctor costume

Some plague doctors wore a special costume, although graphic sources show that plague doctors wore a variety of garments. The garments were invented by Charles de L'Orme in 1619; they were first used in Paris, but later spread to be used throughout Europe.[11] The protective suit consisted of a heavy fabric overcoat that was waxed, a mask with glass eye openings and a cone nose shaped like a beak to hold scented substances and straw.[12]

Some of the scented materials were ambergris, lemon Balm (Melissa officinalis), mint (Mentha spicata L.) leaves, camphor, cloves, laudanum, myrrh, rose petals, storax.[7] This was thought to protect the doctor from miasmatic bad air.[13] The straw provided a filter for the "bad air". A wooden cane pointer was used to help examine the patient without having to touch them. It was also used as a means of repenting sins, as many believed that the plague was a punishment and would ask to be whipped to repent their sins.[14][15]

2.11.3 Public servants

Plague doctors served as public servants during times of epidemics starting with the Black Death of Europe in the fourteenth century. Their principal task, besides taking care of plague victims, was to record in public records the deaths due to the plague.[7]

In certain European cities like Florence and Perugia plague doctors were requested to do autopsies to help determine the cause of death and how the plague played a role.[16] Plague doctors became witnesses to numerous wills during times of plague epidemics.[17] Plague doctors also gave ad-vice to their patients about their conduct before death.[18] This advice varied depending on the patient, and after the Middle Ages the nature of the relationship between doctor and patient was governed by an increasingly complex ethi-cal code.[19]

2.11.4 Methods

Plague doctors practiced bloodletting and other remedies such as putting frogs or leeches on the buboes to "rebalance the humors" as a normal routine.[20] Plague doctors could not generally interact with the general public because of the nature of their business and the possibility of spreading the disease; they could also be subject to quarantine.[21]

2.11.5 Notable medieval plague doctors

A famous plague doctor who gave medical advice about preventive measures which could be against the plague was Nostradamus.[22][23] Nostradamus' advice was the removal of infected corpses, getting fresh air, drinking clean water, and drinking a juice preparation of rose hips.[24][25] In *Traité des fardemens* it shows in Part A Chapter VIII that Nostradamus also recommended *not* to bleed the patient.[25]

The Italian city of Pavia, in 1479, contracted Giovanni de Ventura as a community plague doctor.[5][26] The Irish physician, Niall Ó Glacáin (c.1563?–1653) earned deep respect in Spain, France and Italy for his bravery in treating numerous victims of the plague.[27][28] The French anatomist Ambroise Paré and Paracelsus were also famous medieval plague doctors.[29]

2.11.6 Footnotes

[1] Cipolla, p. 65

[2] Cipolla, p. 68 3/4 down page

[3] Rosenhek, Jackie (October 2011). "Doctors of the Black Death". *Doctor's Review*.

[4] Ellis, p. 202

[5] Byrne (Daily), p. 169

[6] Simon, p. 3

[7] Byrne, 170

[8] Vidal, Pierre; Tibayrenc, Myrtille; Gonzalez, Jean-Paul (2007). "Chapter 40: Infectious disease and arts". In Tibayrenc, Michel. *Encyclopedia of Infectious Diseases: Modern Methodologies*. John Wiley & Sons. p. 680. ISBN 9780470114193.

[9] Gordon, p. 471

[10] Byrne, 168

[11] Christine M. Boeckl, *Images of plague and pestilence: iconography and iconology* (Truman State University Press, 2000), pp. 15, 27.

[12] Byrne (Encyclopedia), p. 505

[13] Irvine Loudon, *Western Medicine: An Illustrated History* (Oxford, 2001), p. 189.

[14] Pommerville, p. 9

[15] O'Donnell, p. 143

[16] Wray, p. 172

[17] Wray, p. 173

[18] "The Plague Doctor". Jhmas.oxfordjournals.org. 2012-04-02. Retrieved 2012-06-12.

[19] Robert S. Gottfried, *The Black Death: natural and human disaster in medieval Europe* (Simon & Schuster, 1983), pp. 126–28.

[20] Byfield, p. 37

[21] Robert S. Gottfried, *The Black Death: natural and human disaster in medieval Europe* (Simon & Schuster, 1983), p. 126.

[22] Hogue, p. 1844

[23] *The essential Nostradamus: literal translation, historical commentary, and ... By Richard Smoley*. Books.google.com. Retrieved 2012-06-12.

[24] Pickover, p. 279

[25] "Excellent et moult utile opuscule à tous/ nécessaire qui désirent avoir connoissan/ ce de plusieurs exquises receptes divisé/ en deux parties./ La première traicte de diverses façons/ de fardemens et senteurs pour illustrer et/ embelir la face./ La seconde nous montre la façon et/ manière de faire confitures de plusieurs/ sortes... Nouvellement composé par Maistre/ Michel de NOSTREDAME docteur/ en medecine... by Nostradamus". Propheties.it. Retrieved 2012-06-12.

[26] King, p. 339

[27] Stephen, p. 927

[28] "THE HISTORY OF MEDICINE IN IRELAND; by J. OLIVER WOODS, MD, FRCGP, Page 40" (PDF). Retrieved 2012-06-12.

[29] Körner, p. 13

2.11.7 References

Primary sources

- Nostradamus. *The Prophecies of Nostradamus*, self-published 1555 & 1558; reprinted by Forgotton Books publishing 1973, ISBN 1-60506-507-2

- Nostradamus. *Traité des fardemens et confitures* self-published 1555

Secondary sources

- Bauer, S. Wise, *The Story of the World Activity Book Two: The Middle Ages : From the Fall of Rome to the Rise of the Renaissance*, Peace Hill Press, 2003, ISBN 0-9714129-4-4

- Byfield, Ted, *Renaissance: God in Man, A.D. 1300 to 1500: But Amid Its Splendors, Night Falls on Medieval Christianity*, Christian History Project, 2010, ISBN 0-9689873-8-9

- Byrne, Joseph Patrick, *Daily Life during the Black Death*, Greenwood Publishing Group, 2006, ISBN 0-313-33297-5

- Byrne, Joseph Patrick, *Encyclopedia of Pestilence, Pandemics, and Plagues*, ABC-Clio, 2008, ISBN 0-313-34102-8

- Cipolla, Carlo M. 'A Plague Doctor', in Harry A. Miskimin *et al.* (eds), *The Medieval City*, Yale University Press, 1977, pp. 65–72. ISBN 0-300-02081-3

- Ellis, Oliver C., *A History of Fire and Flame 1932* , Kessinger Publishing, 2004, ISBN 1-4179-7583-0

- Fee, Elizabeth, *AIDS: the burdens of history*, University of California Press, 1988, ISBN 0-520-06396-1

- Haggard, Howard W., *From Medicine Man to Doctor: The Story of the Science of Healing*, Courier Dover Publications, 2004, ISBN 0-486-43541-5

- Hogue, John,*Nostradamus: the new revelations*, Barnes & Noble Books, 1995, ISBN 1-56619-948-4

- Gordon, Benjamin Lee, *Medieval and Renaissance medicine*, Philosophical Library, 1959

- Heymann, David L., *The World Health Report 2007: a safer future : global public health security in the 21st century*, World Health Organization, 2007, ISBN 92-4-156344-3

- Kenda, Barbara, *Aeolian winds and the spirit in Renaissance architecture: Academia Eolia revisited*, Taylor & Francis, 2006, ISBN 0-415-39804-5

- King, Margaret L., *Western Civilization: a social and cultural history*, Prentice-Hall, 2002, ISBN 0-13-045007-3

- Körner, Christian, *Mountain Biodiversity: a global assessment*, CRC Press, 2002, ISBN 1-84214-091-4

- O'Donnell, Terence, *History of Life Insurance in its Formative Years*, American Conservation Company, 1936

- Pickover, Clifford A., *Dreaming the Future: the fantastic story of prediction*, Prometheus Books, 2001, ISBN 1-57392-895-X

- Pommerville, Jeffrey, *Alcamo's Fundamentals of Microbiology*, Jones & Bartlett Learning, 2010, ISBN 0-7637-6258-X

- Reading, Mario, *The Complete Prophecies of Nostradamus*, Sterling Publishing (2009), ISBN 1-906787-39-5

- Simon, Matthew, *Emergent Computation: emphasizing bioinformatics*, Publisher 　　　　　　　　　　　, 2005, ISBN 0-387-22046-1

- Stuart, David C., *Dangerous Garden: the quest for plants to change our lives*, Frances Lincoln ltd, 2004, ISBN 0-7112-2265-7

- Wray, Shona Kelly, *Communities and Crisis: Bologna during the Black Death*, ISBN 90-04-17634-9

- Fitzharris, Lindsey. "Behind the Mask: The Plague Doctor." The Chirurgeons Apprentice. Web. 6 May 2014.

- Rosenhek, Jackie. "Doctor's Review: Medicine on the Move." Doctor's Review. Web. May 2011.

2.12 Studies of the Fetus in the Womb

Studies of the Fetus in the Womb are two colored annotated sketches by Leonardo da Vinci made in 1510–1512/13. The studies correctly depict the human fetus in its proper position inside the dissected uterus.[1] Da Vinci depicted the uterus with one chamber, in contrast to theories that the uterus had multiple chambers which many believed divided fetuses into separate compartments in the case of twins.[1] Da Vinci also correctly draw the uterine artery and the vascular system of the cervix and vagina.[1]

2.12.1 Preparation and the studies

Da Vinci studied human embryology with the help of anatomist Marcantonio della Torre and saw the fetus within a cadaver.[1] The first study, measuring 30.5×22 cm, shows the fetus in a breech position inside a dissected uterus. Da Vinci mistakenly depicted the cotyledons in the vascular walls of the human uterus that he had previously found in a cow uterus.[2] The other study, measuring 30.3×22 cm, shows female external genitalia, the supposed arrangement of abdominal muscles on the top right and fetus from different angles. The tablet at the top contains an Italian inscription: "Dimanda la moglie di Biagin Crivelli come il cappone alleva le oua della ghallina essendo lui imbricato" ("Ask Biagino Crivelli's wife how the capon rears and hatches the eggs of hens when he is unplucked").[3] Da Vinci theorized that the umbilical cord was responsible for taking the fetus' urine outside of the uterus.[1]

2.12.2 Provenance

The studies were initially bequeathed to Francesco Melzi. In c. 1582–90 they were bought from his heirs by Pompeo Leoni and by 1630 they belonged to Thomas Howard, 2nd Earl of Arundel. Since 1690 the studies are housed in the Royal Collection, United Kingdom.

2.12.3 References

[1] Hilary Gilson. "Leonardo da Vinci's Embryological Drawings of the Fetus". The Embryo Project Encyclopedia. Retrieved 6 Aug 2015.

[2] Leonardo (da Vinci), Kenneth David Keele, Jane Roberts (1983). *Leonardo Da Vinci: Anatomical Drawings from the Royal Library, Windsor Castle*. Metropolitan Museum of Art. p. 78. ISBN 0870993623.

[3] *Leonardo Da Vinci: Anatomical Drawings from the Royal Library, Windsor Castle*, p. 75

2.12.4 External links

- Royal Collection entry

2.13 Unani medicine

Yunani or *Unani* medicine (Urdu: طب یونانی *tibb yūnānī*[1]) is the term for Perso-Arabic traditional medicine as practiced in Mughal India and in Muslim culture in South Asia. The term is derived from Arabic *Yūnānī* "Greek", as the Perso-Arabic system of medicine was in turn based on the teachings of the Greek physicians Hippocrates and Galen.[2]

The Hellenistic origin of Unani medicine is still visible in its being based on the classical four humours: Phlegm (Balgham), Blood (Dam), Yellow bile (Ṣafrā') and Black bile (Saudā'), but it has also been influenced by Indian and Chinese traditional systems.[3]

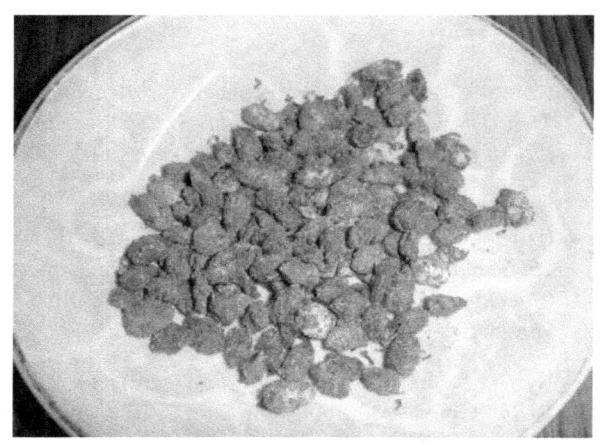
Birbahuti (Trombidium) is used as Unani Medicine

2.13.1 History

Further information: Medicine in the medieval Islamic world

Unani medicine is substantially based on Ibn Sina's *The Canon of Medicine* (11th century).[4]

The medical tradition of medieval Islam was introduced to India by the 13th century with the establishment of the Delhi Sultanate and it took its own course of development during the Mughal Empire,[5][6] influenced by Indian medical teachings of Sushruta and Charaka.[7][8] Alauddin Khilji (d. 1316) had several eminent physicians (Hakims) at his royal courts.[9] This royal patronage meant development of Unani practice in India, but also of Unani literature with the aid of Indian Ayurvedic physicians.[10][11]

2.13.2 Diagnosis and treatment

Unani classical literature consists of thousands of books. According to Unani medicine, management of any disease depends upon the diagnosis of disease. In the diagnosis, clinical features, i.e., signs, symptoms, laboratory features and mizaj (temperament) are important.

Any cause and or factor is countered by Quwwat-e-Mudabbira-e-Badan (the power of body responsible to maintain health), the failing of which may lead to quantitatively or qualitatively derangement of the normal equilibrium of akhlat (humors) of body which constitute the tissues and organs. This abnormal humor leads to pathological changes in the tissues anatomically and physiologically at the affected site and exhibits the clinical manifestations.

After diagnosing the disease, Usoole Ilaj (principle of management) of disease is determined on the basis of etiology

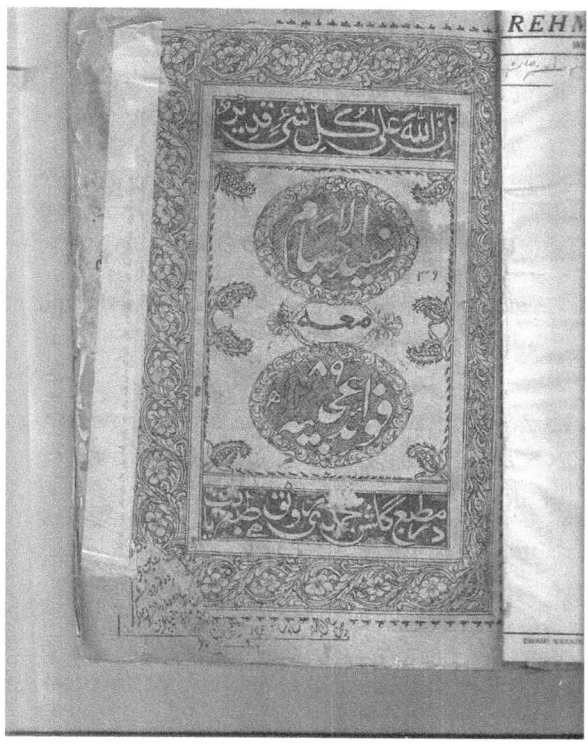

A title page of Unani book on physiology in Urdu Language printed in 1289 Hijri(1868 AD) in India

in the following pattern:

Izalae Sabab (elimination of cause)

Tadeele Akhlat (normalization of humors)

Tadeele Aza (normalization of tissues/organs)

For fulfillment of requirements of principle of management, treatment is decided as per the Unani medicine which may be one or more of the following:

- Ilaj-Bil-Tadbeer wa Ilaj-Bil-Ghiza (Regimenal Therapy). The disease may be treated by the modification of six essential pre-requisites of health (Asbab-e-Sitta Zarooriya in Unani Tibbi terminology). Asbab-e-Sitta Zarooriya may be modified by the use of one or more regimens: i.e., Dalak, Riyazat, Hammam, Taleeq, Takmeed, Hijamat (Cupping Therapy), Fasd, Lakhlakha, Bakhur, Abzan, Shamoomat (Aromatherapy), Pashoya, Idrar, Ishal, Qai, Tareeq, Elam, Laza-e-Muqabil, Imalah and

alteration of food. According to the norms of C.C.I.M. New Delhi, Department of Ilaj-Bil-Tadbeer has been established in almost all Unani Tibbi Colleges of India. In the State Unani Medical College, Allahabad, U.P. and State Takmeel-Ul-Tibb College, Lucknow, Department of Ilaj-Bil-Tadbeer is known as Moalijat Khususi. Moaliajt Khususi is the old nomenclature of Ilaj-Bil-Tadbeer, suggested by C.C.I.M. New Delhi. Ilaj-Bil-Tadbeer is synonym to Panchkarma in Ayurveda.

- Ilaj-Bil-Advia (Pharmacotherapy). For this purpose Mamulate Matab Nuskha (prescription) is formulated which contain the single and or compound (murakkābāt) Unani drugs[12] having desired actions as per requirements.

- Ilaj-Bil-Yad (Surgery)

As an alternative form of medicine, Unani has found favor in India where popular products like Roghan Baiza Murgh (Egg Oil) and Roghan Badaam Shirin (Almond Oil) are commonly used for hair care. Unani practitioners can practice as qualified doctors in India, as the government approves their practice. Unani medicine has similarities to Ayurveda. Both are based on theory of the presence of the elements (in Unani, they are considered to be fire, water, earth and air) in the human body. (The elements, attributed to the philosopher Empedocles, determined the way of thinking in Medieval Europe.) According to followers of Unani medicine, these elements are present in different fluids and their balance leads to health and their imbalance leads to illness.

The theory postulates the presence of blood, phlegm, yellow bile and black bile in the human body. Each person's unique mixture of these substances determines his Mizaj (temperament). a predominance of blood gives a sanguine temperament; a predominance of phlegm makes one phlegmatic; yellow bile, bilious (or choleric); and black bile, melancholic.

2.13.3 Education and recognition

In India, there are 40 Unani medical colleges where the Unani system of medicine is taught. After five and half year courses, the graduates are awarded BUMS (Bachelor of Unani Medicine and Surgery). There are about eight Unani medical colleges where a postgraduate degree (Mahir-e-Tib and Mahir Jarahat) is being awarded to BUMS doctors. All these colleges are affiliated to reputed universities and recognized by the governments.

In India, the Central Council of Indian Medicine (CCIM) a statutory body established in 1971 under Department of Ayurveda, Yoga and Naturopathy, Unani, Siddha and Homoeopathy (AYUSH), Ministry of Health and Family Welfare, Government of India, monitors higher education in areas of Indian medicine including, Ayurveda, Unani and Siddha.[13] To fight biopiracy and unethical patents, the Government of India, in 2001, set up the Traditional Knowledge Digital Library as repository of formulations of systems of Indian medicine, includes 98,700 Unani formulations.[14][15] Central Council for Research in Unani Medicine (CCRUM)[16] established in 1979, also under AYUSH, aids and co-ordinates scientific research in the Unani system of medicine through a network of 22 nationwide research institutes and units, including two Central Research Institutes of Unani Medicine, at Hyderabad and Lucknow, eight Regional Research Institutes at Chennai, Bhadrak, Patna, Aligarh, Mumbai, Srinagar, Kolkata and New Delhi, six Clinical Research Units at Allahabad, Bangalore, Karimganj, Meerut, Bhopal and Burhanpur, four Drug Standardisation Research Units at New Delhi, Bangalore, Chennai and Lucknow, a Chemical Research Unit at Aligarh, a Literary Research Institute at New Delhi.[17]

In Pakistan, National Council for Tibb, Govt.of Pakistan is awarding four years Fazil-ut-Tibb-wal-Jarahat (B.U.M.S) and registration certificates to every 4 years qualified Tabibs/Unani Physicians, Doctors. Hamdard Foundation and Qarshi Foundation are prominent patrons of research and development in herbal medicines. Hamdard Research Institute of Unani Medicine at the Hamdard University offers advance degrees in the field.[18] The programs are accredited by Higher Education Commission (HEC),[19] Pakistan Medical and Dental Council (PMDC),[20] and the Pakistan Pharmacy Council (PCP).[21]

The Department of Eastern Medicine and Surgery at Qarshi University, Pakistan offers education and training in a network of clinics and dispensaries across the country under Qarshi Foundation so that students acquire clinical skills under the guidance of experienced *Hakeem* during their academic training.[22]

Qarshi Industries, Pakistan is one of the leading pharmaceutical companies manufacturing products using Ayurveda and Unani system of medicines.

2.13.4 Safety issues

The Indian Journal of Pharmacology notes:

> According to WHO, "Pharmacovigilance activities are done to monitor detection, assessment, understanding and prevention of any obnoxious adverse reactions to drugs at therapeutic concentration that is used or is intended to be used to modify or explore physiological system or pathological states for the benefit of recipient." These drugs may be any substance or product including herbs, minerals, etc. for animals and human beings and can even be that prescribed by practitioners of **Unani** or ayurvedic system of medicine. In recent days, awareness has been created related to safety and adverse drug reaction monitoring of herbal drugs including Unani drugs.[23]

2.13.5 Notable Unani organizations/institutions

- Hamdard Al-Majeed College of Eastern Medicine, Hamdard University, Pakistan

- Central Research Institute of Unani Medicine, Hyderabad

- Ibn Sina Academy of Medieval Medicine and Sciences, India.

- National Institute of Unani Medicine, Bangalore, (Government of India)

- Tipu Sultan Unani Medical College, Gulbarga, Karnataka.

- Govt. Unani and Ayurvedic Medical College & Hospital, Dhaka, Bangladesh

2.13.6 See also

- Ayurveda

- Yoga and Naturopathy

- Siddha medicine

- Sowa Rigpa

- Dawakhana Shifaul Amraz

- Hakim Abdul Aziz

- Hakim Ajmal Khan

- Hakim Habibur Rahman

- Hakim Hammad Usmani

- Hakim Mohammed Said

- Hakim Syed Atiqul Qadir

- Hakim Syed Fazlur Rahman

- Hakim Syed Karam Husain

- Hakim Syed Zillur Rahman

- Hamdard (Wakf) Laboratories

- Hamdard Laboratories (Waqf)

- Qazi Mazhar Qayyum

- Traditional Knowledge Digital Library

2.13.7   References

[1] the transcription as *Unani* is found in 19th-century English language sources: "the *Ayurvedic* and *Unani* systems of medicine" "Madhya Pradesh District Gazetteers: Hoshangabad", *Gazetteer of India* 17 (1827), p. 587.

[2] Unani Medicine in India: Its Origin and Fundamental Concepts by Hakim Syed Zillur Rahman, History of Science, Philosophy and Culture in Indian Civilization, Vol. IV Part 2 (Medicine and Life Sciences in India), Ed. B. V. Subbarayappa, Centre for Studies in Civilizations, Project of History of Indian Science, Philosophy and Culture, New Delhi, 2001, pp. 298-325

[3] "The use of Chinese herbal drugs in Islamic medicine". *Journal of Integrative Medicine.*   doi:10.1016/S2095-4964(15)60205-9.

[4] Unani Medicine in India during 1901–1947 by Hakim Syed Zillur Rahman, Studies in History of Medicine and Science, IHMMR, New Delhi, Vol. XIII, No. 1, 1994, p. 97-112. Arab Medicine during the Ages by Hakim Syed Zillur Rahman, Studies in History of Medicine and Science, IHMMR, New Delhi, Vol. XIV, No. 1-2, 1996, p. 1-39

[5] Chishti, p. 2.

[6] Kapoor, p. 7264

[7] Exchanges between India and Central Asia in the field of Medicine by Hakeem Abdul Hameed

[8] Interaction with China and Central Asia in the Field of Unani Medicine by Hakim Syed Zillur Rahman, History of Science, Philosophy and Culture in Indian Civilization, Vol. III Part 2 (India's Interaction with China, Central and West Asia), Ed. A. Rahman, Centre for Studies in Civilizations, Project of History of Indian Science, Philosophy and Culture, New Delhi, 2002, pp. 297-314

[9] Indian Hakims: Their Role in the medical care of India by Hakim Syed Zillur Rahman, History of Science, Philosophy and Culture in Indian Civilization, Vol. IV Part 2 (Medicine and Life Sciences in India), Ed. B. V. Subbarayappa, Centre for Studies in Civilizations, Project of History of Indian Science, Philosophy and Culture, New Delhi, 2001, pp. 371-426

[10] "Unani". Department of Ayurveda, Yoga and Naturopathy, Unani, Siddha and Homoeopathy, Govt. of India.

[11] Bala, p. 45

[12] Hakim Syed Zillur Rahman (1980), *Kitāb al-murakkabāt*, ʻAlīgaṛh: Pablikeshan Ḍivīzhan, Muslim Yūnivarsiṭī

[13] CCIM

[14] Traditional Knowledge Digital Library website.

[15] "Know Instances of Patenting on the UES of Medicinal Plants in India". PIB, Ministry of Environment and Forests. May 6, 2010.

[16] "Central Council for Research in Unani Medicine (CCRUM)". Traditional Knowledge Digital Library.

[17] "Research and Development: Central Council for Research in Unani Medicine (CCRUM)". Centre for Research in Indian Systems of Medicine, (CRISM).

[18] "Hamdard Research Institute of Unani Medicine, Hamdard University". Retrieved 11 January 2015.

[19] "H.E.C. Accreditation List".

[20] "PM&DC Accreditation List". Retrieved 2012-08-03.

[21] "PCP Accreditation List". Pharmacy Council of Pakistan. Retrieved 2013-02-19.

[22] "Department of Eastern Medicine and Surgery, Qarshi University". Retrieved 11 January 2015.

[23] Rahman, SZ; Latif, A; Khan, RA (Dec 2008). "Importance of pharmacovigilance in Unani system of medicine". *Indian J Pharmacol.* **40** (7): 17–20.

2.13.8   Further reading

- *Standardisation of single drugs of Unani medicine.* Central Council for Research in Unani Medicine (India), Ministry of Health and Family Welfare, Govt. of India, 1987.

- *Unani: the science of Graeco-Arabic medicine*, by Jamil Ahmad, Hakim Ashhar Qadeer. Lustre Press, 1998. ISBN 81-7436-052-2.

- *The Unani Pharmacopoeia of India*, Dept. of Indian Systems of Medicine & Homoeopathy. Pub. Govt. of India, Ministry of Health & Family Welfare, Dept. of Indian Systems of Medicine & Homoeopathy, 1999.

- *Physicochemical standards of Unani formulations*, Pub. Central Council for Research in Unani Medicine, Ministry of Health & Family Welfare, Govt. of India, 2006.

- Hakim Syed Zillur Rahman (1986), *Qānūn-i ibn-i Sīnā aur us ke shārḥīn va mutarajimīn*, ʿAlīgaṛh: Pablīkeshan Dīvīzan, Muslim Yūnīvarsiṭī

- *Refiguring unani tibb: plural healing in late colonial India*, by Guy N. A. Attewell. Orient Longman, 2007. ISBN 81-250-3017-4.

- *Hand book on unani medicines with formulae, processes, uses and analysis*. National Institute Of Industrial Research, 2008. ISBN 81-7833-042-3.

- Chishti, Hakim (1990). *The traditional healer's handbook: a classic guide to the medicine of Avicenna*. Inner Traditions / Bear & Company. ISBN 0-89281-438-1.

- Kapoor, Subodh (2002). *The Indian encyclopaedia. Archery-Banog, Volume 2*. Genesis Publishing. ISBN 81-7755-257-0.

- Bala, Poonam (2007). *Medicine and medical policies in India: social and historical perspectives*. Lexington Books. ISBN 0-7391-1322-4.

- 10 Unani medicine books online at Traditional Knowledge Digital Library (Govt. of India)

- Hakim Syed Zillur Rahman (1995), *Dillī aur ṭibb-i Yūnānī* (Dillī aur ṭibb-i Yūnānī ed.), Naʾī Dihlī: Urdū Akādmī, Dihlī

- Hakim Syed Zillur Rahman (1962), *Daur-e Jadeed aur Tib*, Bhopal, India: Tibbi Academy, India

- Hakim Syed Zillur Rahman (1983), *Ṣafvī ʿahd meṉ ʿilm-i tashrīḥ kā muṭālaʿah*, ʿAlīgaṛh: Ṭibbī Akādmī

2.13.9 External links

- Directory of History of Medicine Collection

2.14 Unicorn horn

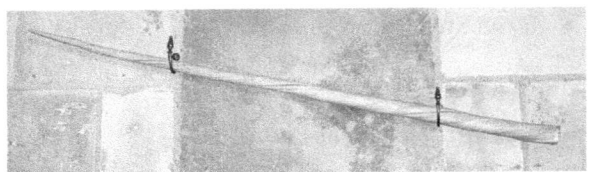

Narwhal tooth presented as a unicorn horn.

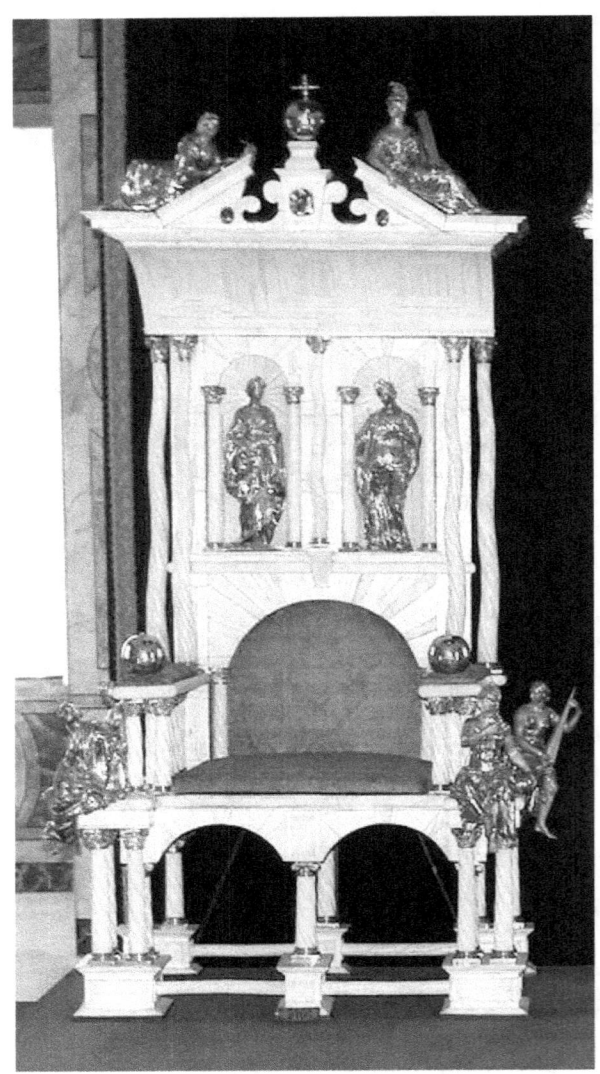

The unicorn throne in Denmark.

"Alicorn" redirects here. In some literature and media, "alicorn" refers to a winged unicorn.

A **unicorn horn**, also known as an **alicorn**,[1] is a legendary object whose reality may have been accepted in Western Europe throughout the Middle Ages. Many healing powers and antidote's virtues were attributed to the horn of the unicorn. These properties, assumed real since the 13th century, made it one of the most expensive and most reputable remedies during the Renaissance,[2] and justified its use in royal courts. Beliefs related to the "unicorn horn" influenced alchemy through spagyric medicine. The horn's purification properties were eventually put to the test in, for example, the book of Ambroise Paré, *Discourse on unicorn* - marking the beginnings of the experimental method.

Seen as one of the most valuable assets that a king could possess, unicorn horns were exchanged and could be purchased at apothecaries as universal antidotes until the 18th century. Other horns were displayed in cabinets of curiosities. The horn was used to create sceptres and other royal objects, such as the "unicorn throne" of the Danish kings, the sceptre and imperial crown of the Austrian Empire, and the scabbard and the hilt of the sword of Charles the Bold. The legendary unicorn was never captured, but its symbolic association with virginity made it the symbol of the incarnation of God's Word, innocence and divine power

Belief in the power of the unicorn's horn and its origins persisted from the Middle Ages to the 18th century, when the true source, the narwhal, was discovered. This marine mammal is the true bearer of the "unicorn horn", actually an extended tooth found in the mouth of males and some females. Since then, the unicorn horn has been mentioned in fantasy works, role-playing games and video games, which make use of its legendary symbolism.

2.14.1 Nature and properties

Coming from an ancient figure, the unicorn was described by Ctesias as carrying a horn which Indian princes would use to make hanaps against poison. These writings were taken up by Aristotle and Pliny the Elder;[3] Claudius Aelianus also said that drinking in this horn protects against diseases and poisons.[4] These writings influenced the authors from the Middle Ages to the Renaissance: the unicorn becomes the most important and most frequently mentioned imaginary animal in the West, its existence was considered real. Other parts of its body were given medicinal properties and, in the 12th century, abbess Hildegard of Bingen recommended an ointment against leprosy made from foie de licorne and egg yolk.[5] Wearing a unicorn leather belt was supposed to protect a person from the plague and fever, while leather shoes of this animal lure diseases away from feet.[6]

The actual medicinal use was linked to its horn and purification power assumed true since the Antiquity, which was explicitly mentioned for the first time in the 13th century. Legends about this properties circulating since the Middle Ages were are the origin of a flourishing trade of these objects, which became more common up to the late 18th century, when their true origin was unknown. The unicorn never existed as represented, it is most often narwhal teeth known as "unicorn horns" during these times.[7]

Water purification

The first reference to the cleansing power of the unicorn appears in an interpretation of the *Physiologus* (dated 14th century), when reference is made to a large lake where animals congregate to drink:

> But before they are gathered, the snake comes
> and throws his poison in the water. So many ani-

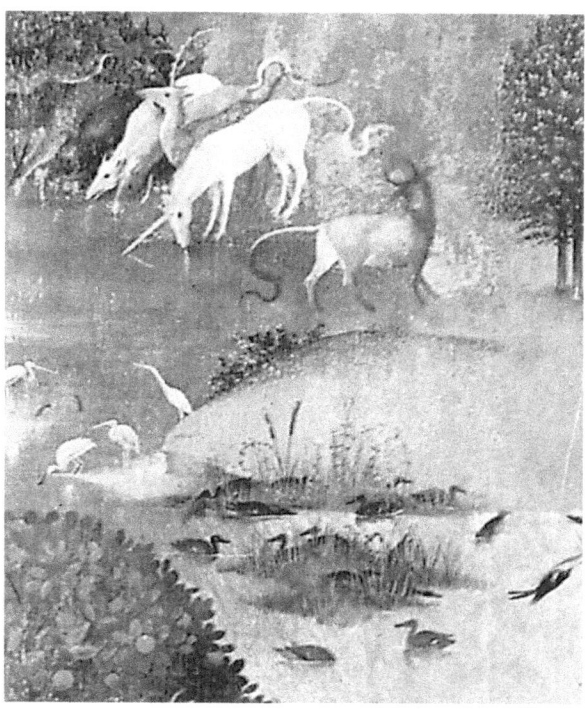

Left panel of The Garden of Earthly Delights *by Hieronymus Bosch (1503-1504), showing unicorns purifying water.*

mals notice the poison and dare not to drink, and they expect the unicorn. It comes and it goes immediately to the lake, with its horn making the sign of the cross, it makes the poison harmless. All other animals drink then.[8]

The theme soon became popular, the stage of purification of water by a unicorn is taken in 1389 by the father Johann van Hesse, who claims to have seen a unicorn emerge from the sea to clean impure water so that animals could drink[9] Symbolically, the snake that poisons the water is the devil and the unicorn represent Christ the Redeemer.[10] The origin of this legend seems Indian, through the Greek texts mention the fact that the Indian nobles might drink out of unicorn horns to protect themselves from diseases and poisons.[9]

The unicorn is most often represented by a river, a lake or a fountain, while animals wait for her to finish her work to drink. This scene is very common in the art of the 16th and 17th centuries.[11] Studies and translations of these drawings and stories popularized the belief that the power of the animal comes from its horn, which would eliminate the poisons as it hits a liquid.[9] Water purification forge the legend on the properties of the "unicorn horn" and later justifies its use as a universal antidote.

Medicinal properties

See also: Bezoar

The properties of the unicorn horn can be paralleled to

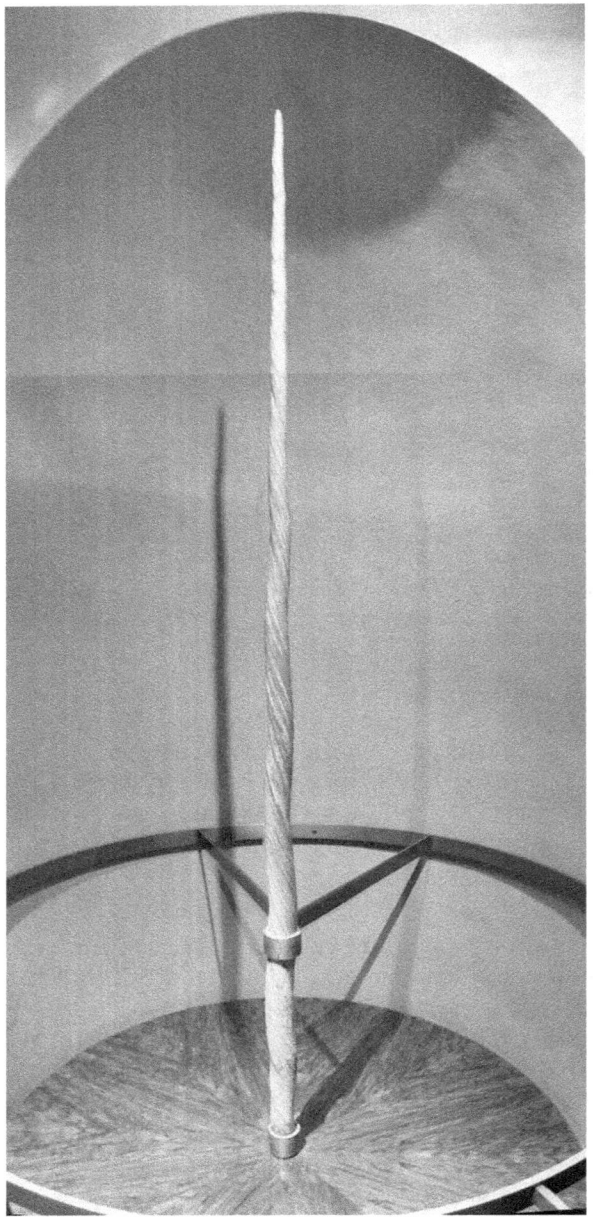

Ainkhürn, «unicorn horn», offered to the Holy Roman Emperor Ferdinand I in 1540, exposed at Wiener Schatzkammer.

those of the bezoar stone, another object of animal origin known in the Renaissance medicine and exposed as a rarity in the cabinets of curiosities.[12]

The unicorn horn was very quickly assigned many medicinal properties and, over time, in addition to the purification of polluted water in nature,[13] its use was recommended against rubella, measles, fevers and pains.[14] The monks of the Parisians monasteries used to soak it in the drinking water given to lepers.[13] It acted as an antidote and, in a powder form, was known to facilitate wound healing, help neutralize poisons (such as scorpion or viper venom)[15] or against the plague.[16] It would also have an aphrodisiac power known since ancient times[17] and would test the virginity of young girls.[18] The horn was consumed in several ways, in substance or infusion[19]

Its prophylactic function and magical power, although known for centuries, while its trade increases, several «fake» horns and false powders appeared.[20] The astronomical value achieved by these objects left to assume that their imaginary virtues could cause real healing,[13] probably due to the placebo effect.

This use of the unicorn horn in medicine is due to the fact that therapists then have very few instruments and objects, and the ancient heritage meant that they were only instruments of God. The Inquisition played a role in this belief: to doubt the powers of the horn meant doubting the existence of the unicorn itself, animal of God mentioned in a translation of the Bible. Skeptics risked to be burned at the stake.[21]

Many works are devoted to the explanation and defense of the medicinal properties of the «unicorn horn», including *The Treaty of the Unicorn, its wonderful properties and its use* (1573) by Andrea Bacci and *Natural History, Hunting, Virtues, and Use of Lycorn* (1624) by apothecary Laurent Catelan. Bacci probably wrote his book at the request of his patients, who were major investors in the unicorn horn trade.[22]

Display and use as antipoison

Twisted shape "unicorn horns" were exchanged and in circulation for a long time: according to a legend, the "horn" on display at the Musée national du Moyen Âge was a gift from the Caliph of Baghdad, Harun al-Rashid, to Charlemagne in 807.[4] It measures almost three meters.[23] An eight-foot long horn is exposed in Bruges, Flanders.[4] Since the Middle Ages, the "unicorn horn" is supposed to be the most valuable asset that a king could possess.[15] Its medicinal use is attested since the 13th century, when pharmacists incorporated narwhal teeth (presented as unicorn horns) in their treatments and they had large pieces so it could not be confused with that of another animal, such as ox.[24] These objects would have been exchanged up to eleven times their weight in gold.[13] Some horns, introduced reportedly during the Fourth Crusade of Constantinople, were thrown into the pit of the Doge's Palace in Venice, so that water could never be poisoned. Horns considered sacred relics can be found at the Council of Trent in 1563, as well as the Saint-Denis Cathedral in Paris, St Mark's Basilica in Venice and Westminster Abbey in London. They were usually mounted on silver socles and presented as trophies that could only be shown for important ceremonies.[15]

Ambroise Paré explains that the horns were used in the court of the King of France to detect the presence of poison in food and drink: if the horn became hot and started to smoke, then the dish was poisoned.[25] Pope Clement VII would have offered a unicorn horn of two cubits long to King Francis I of France at the wedding of his niece Catherine de' Medici in Marseille in October 1533,[26] and the king did not ever move without a bag filled with unicorn powder.[3] Also, the Grand Inquisitor Torquemada always bore his unicorn horn to protect himself from poison and murderers.[27]

2.14.2 References

[1] Shepard, Odell (1930). *The Lore of the Unicorn*. London: Unwin and Allen. ISBN 9781437508536.

[2] (Faidutti 1996, p. 13)

[3] (Davenne 2004, p. 130)

[4] (de Tervarent 1997, pp. 281–287)

[5] (de Bingen 1989, pp. 196–197)

[6] (Lecouteux 1993, p. 45)

[7] Didrit, Mireille; Pujol, Raymond (September 1996). "Note de recherche d'Ethnozoologie : Licorne de Mer ou Licorne de Terre : le Narval" (in French). Paris: Université Paris V - Sorbonne. Retrieved 21 September 2012.

[8] *Der Physiologus* cited in (Freeman 1983, p. 27)

[9] (Faidutti 1996, p. 39)

[10] (Faidutti 1996, p. 59)

[11] (Faidutti 1996, p. 61)

[12] Martin, Jean Hubert; Jean Guillaume and Frédéric Didier (2000). *Le château d'Oiron et son cabinet de curiosités*. Éditions du patrimoine, p. 131

[13] (Rochelandet 2003, p. 131)

[14] (Valentini 1704, p. vol. 3, ch. 30)

[15] (Brasey 2007, pp. 259–263)

[16] Paré, Ambroise (1628). *Les œuvres d'Ambroise Paré* (in French). N. Buon. p. 812. Retrieved September 28, 2012.

[17] (Ferlampin-Acher 2002, p. 297)

[18] Graitson, Jean-Marie (1997). *Actes du colloque Frankenstein littérature/cinéma*. Chaudfontaine. p. 68. ISBN 9782871300540. Retrieved September 28, 2012.

[19] (Pomet 1696, p. 26)

[20] (Rochelandet 2003, p. 130)

[21] (Lemoine 1996, p. 147)

[22] (Giblin 1991, p. 77)

[23] Mireille Didrit and Raymond Pujol (1996). *Licorne de Mer ou Licorne de Terre : le Narval* (Master). Université Paris-V - Sorbonne.

[24] (Buck & Centre d'études supérieures de la Renaissance 1973, p. 215)

[25] (Malrieu 1987, p. 131)

[26] Fagnart, Laure (2009). *Léonard de Vinci en France: collections et collectionneurs : XVe-XVIIe siècles* (in French). L'Erma di Bretschneider. p. 161. ISBN 9788882655549.

[27] (Lutavd 1906, pp. 197–199)

2.14.3 Bibliography

Founding works on medicine and alchemy

- de Bingen, Hildegarde (1989). *Le Livre des subtilités des créatures divines* (in French) **II**. Paris: Millon. ISBN 2905614315.

- Marini, Andrea (1566). *Discorso contro la falsa opinione dell'Alicorno* (in Italian). Venice.

- Bacci, Andrea (1573). *L'alicorno discorso dell'eccellente medico et filosofo M. Andrea Bacci: nel quale si tratta della natura dell' alicorno et delle sue virtu eccellentissime* (in Italian). G. Marescotti. p. 80.

- Paré, Ambroise (1582). *Discours d'Ambroise Paré : À savoir, de la mumie, de la licorne, des venins et de la peste* (in French). Paris. Retrieved September 20, 2012.

- Paré, Ambroise (1928). *Voyages et apologie suivis du Discours de la licorne* (in French).

- Pomis, David (1587). *Dittionario novo hebraïco* (in Italian). Venice.

- Linocier, Geoffroy (1584). *Histoire des plantes avec leurs pourtraictz, à laquelle sont adjoutées celles des simples, aromatiques, animaux à quatre pieds, oiseaux, serpens et autres bêtes venimeuses* (in French). Paris. Retrieved September 20, 2012.

- Valentine, Basil (1678). *Triumphal Chariot of Antimony*. Retrieved September 20, 2012.

- Rodrigo a Castro, Esteban (1621). *De Meteoris Microcosmi* (in Italian). Florence.

- Catelan, Laurent (1624). *Histoire de la nature, chasse, vertus, proprietez et usage de la lycorne* (in French).

- Pomet, Pierre (1696). *Histoire générale des drogues, traitant des plantes, des minéraux et des animaux* (in French) **II**. Paris. Retrieved September 20, 2012.

Founding travel and exploration stories

- Belon, Pierre (1553). *Les Observations de plusieurs singularités et choses mémorables trouvées en Grèce, Asie, Judée, Égypte, Arabie et autres pays estranges, rédigées en trois livres* (in French). Paris: G. Corrozet.

- Goropius, Johannes (1569). *Origines Antwerpianæ* (in Dutch). Antwerp.

- Mercator, Gérard (1607). *Atlas Minor: traduction française par M. de la Popelinière* (in French). Amsterdam.

- Bartholin, Thomas (1645). *De Unicornu Observationes Novæ* (in Latin). Padoue. Retrieved September 20, 2012.

- Collinson, Sir Richard (1867). *The Three Voyages of Martin Frobisher in Search of a Passage to Cathaia and India by the North-West, 1576-8, A.D. 1576-8*. London: Hakluyt Society. p. 374. Retrieved September 20, 2012.

Founding works on zoology

- Gesner, Conrad (1603). *Historiæ Animalium de Quadrupedibus Viviparis* (in Latin). Frankfurt. Retrieved September 20, 2012.

- Aldrovandi, Ulysse (1616). *De Quadrupedibus Solipedibus* (in Italian). Bologna. Retrieved September 20, 2012.

- Valentini, Michael Bernhard (1704). "30". *Museum Museorum* (in Latin) **III**. Frankfurt.

- von Linné, Carl (1793). *Systema Naturae* (in Latin). Brussels.

Theses and studies

- Faidutti, Bruno (1996). *Images et connaissance de la licorne: (Fin du Moyen Âge - xixe siècle)* (Ph.D.) (in French) **1**. Université Paris-XII. Retrieved 10 June 2009.

- Freeman, Margaret (1983). *La chasse à la licorne: prestigieuse tenture française des Cloisters* (in French). Lausanne: Edita. p. 247. ISBN 9782880010508.

- Lecouteux, Claude (1993). *Les monstres dans la pensée médiévale européenne: essai de présentation* (in French). Paris: Presses de l'Université de Paris-Sorbonne. p. 183. ISBN 9782840500216.

- de Tervarent, Guy (1997). *Attributs et symboles dans l'art profane: dictionnaire d'un langage perdu (1450-1600)* (in French). Librairie Droz. p. 535. ISBN 9782600005074. Retrieved September 20, 2012.

- Davenne, Christine (2004). *Modernité du cabinet de curiosités* (in French). L'Harmattan. p. 299. ISBN 9782747558600. Retrieved September 20, 2012.

External links

- The dictionary definition of alicorn at Wiktionary

Chapter 3

Islamic Medicine during the Medieval Period

3.1 Bimaristan

See also: Medicine in the medieval Islamic world

Bimaristan is a Persian word (بیمارستان *bīmārestān*) meaning "hospital", with *Bimar-* from Middle Persian (Pahlavi) of *vīmār* or *vemār*, meaning "sick" plus *-stan* as location and place suffix. In the medieval Islamic world, the word "Bimaristan" was used to indicate a hospital where the ill were welcomed and cared for by qualified staff.

3.1.1 See also

- Academy of Gondishapur

- Dar al-Shifa

- Medicine in the medieval Islamic world

3.1.2 Further reading

- Morelon, Régis; Rashed, Roshdi (1996), *Encyclopedia of the History of Arabic Science* **3**, Routledge, ISBN 0-415-12410-7

- Noshwrawy, A.R., *The Islamic Biarmistans in the Middle Ages*, Arabic Translation by M. Kh. Badra, The Arab Legacy Bul. No. 21, P 202

3.2 Byzantine medicine

Byzantine medicine encompasses the common medical practices of the Byzantine Empire from about 400 AD to 1453 AD. Byzantine medicine was notable for building upon the knowledge base developed by its Greco-Roman predecessors. In preserving medical practices from antiquity, Byzantine medicine influenced Islamic medicine as well as fostering the Western rebirth of medicine during the Renaissance.

Byzantine physicians often compiled and standardized medical knowledge into textbooks. Their records tended to include both diagnostic explanations and technical drawings. The Medical Compendium in Seven Books, written by the leading physician Paul of Aegina, survived as a particularly thorough source of medical knowledge. This compendium, written in the late seventh century, remained in use as a standard textbook for the following 800 years.

Late antiquity ushered in a revolution in medical science, and historical records often mention civilian hospitals (although battlefield medicine and wartime triage were recorded well before Imperial Rome). Constantinople stood out as a center of medicine during the Middle Ages, which was aided by its crossroads location, wealth, and accumulated knowledge.

3.2.1 Background

Arguably, the first Byzantine physician was the author of the Vienna Dioscurides manuscript, created circa 515 AD for the daughter of Emperor Olybrius. Like most Byzantine physicians, this author drew his material from ancient authorities like Galen and Hippocrates, though Byzantine doctors expanded upon the knowledge preserved from Greek and Roman sources. Oribasius, arguably the most prolific Byzantine compiler of medical knowledge, frequently made note of standing medical assumptions that were proved incorrect. Several of his works, along with those of other Byzantine physicians, were translated into Latin, and eventually, during the Enlightenment and Age of Reason, into English and French.

Another Byzantine treatise, that of the thirteenth century doctor Nicholas Myrepsos, remained the principal pharmaceutical code of the Parisian medical faculty until 1651, while the Byzantine tract of Demetrios Pepagomenos (thirteenth century) on gout was translated and published in Latin by the post-Byzantine humanist Marcus Musurus, in Venice in 1517. Therefore it could be argued that previous misrepresentations about Byzantium being simply a 'carrier' of Ancient Medical knowledge to the Renaissance are wrong. It is known, for example, that the late twelfth-century Italian physician (Roger of Salerno) was influenced by the treatises of the Byzantine doctors Aëtius and Alexander of Tralles as well as Paul of Aegina.

The last great Byzantine physician was John Actuarius, who lived in the early 14th Century in Constantinople. His works on urine laid much of the foundation for later study in urology. However, from the latter 12th Century to the fall of Constantinople to the Turks in 1453, there was very little further dissemination of medical knowledge, largely due to the turmoil the Empire was facing on both fronts, following its resurrection after the Latin Empire and the dwindling population of Constantinople due to plague and war. Nevertheless, Byzantine medicine is extremely important both in terms of new discoveries made in that period (at a time when Western Europe was in turmoil), the collection of ancient Greek and Roman knowledge, and its dissemination to both Renaissance Italy and the Islamic world.

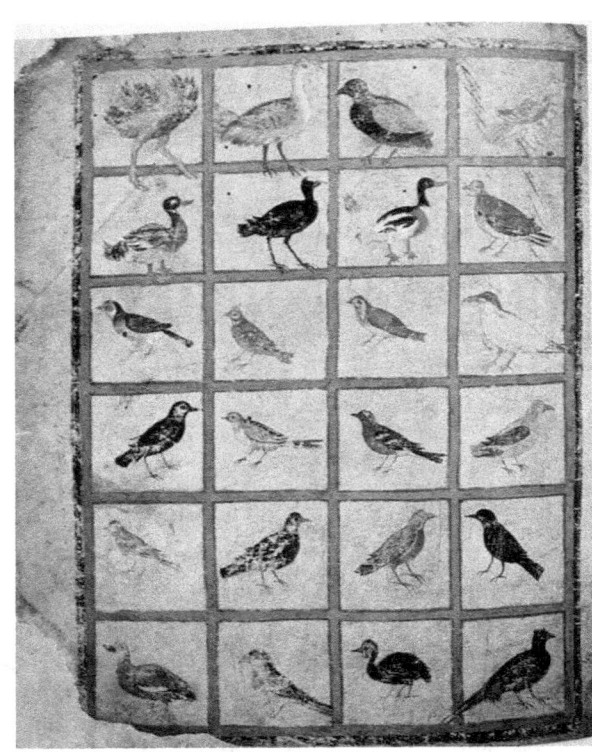

A gallery of birds from the Vienna Dioscurides Byzantine manuscript.

3.2.2 Hospitals

Byzantium was the first empire in which dedicated medical establishments flourished. These were usually set up by individual churches or the state and parallel modern hospitals in many ways. Although similar establishments existed in Ancient Greece and Rome, they differed in that they were usually either institutions for military use, or hospices where citizens went to die in a more peaceful way. Medical institutions of this sort were common in imperial cities such as Constantinople and later Thessaloniki.

The first hospital was built by Basil of Caesarea in the late a.d. 4th century, and although these institutions thrived, it was only throughout the 8th and 9th centuries that they began to appear in provincial towns as well as cities, (although Justinian's subsidization of private physicians to work publicly for six months of the year can be seen as the real breakthrough point). Byzantine medicine was based around hospitals or walk-in dispensaries which formed part of a hospital complex. There was a hierarchy of roles, including the chief physician (*archiatroi*), professional nurses (*hypourgoi*) and orderlies (*hyperetai*).

Doctors themselves were well trained; some attended the University of Constantinople, as medicine had become a scholarly subject by the period of Byzantium (despite the prominence of the great physicians of antiquity, its sta-

tus as a science was greatly improved through its application in formal education (particularly in the University of Constantinople). This rigidity through professionalism (similar to the professionalism exhibited in the Byzantine bureaucracy) bears many hallmarks of today's modern hospitals, and many comparisons are made by modern scholars studying this field. Thus, we know that in the 12th century, Constantinople had two well organized hospitals staffed by medical specialists (including women doctors), with special wards for various types of diseases and systematic methods of treatment.

3.2.3 Christianity

Christianity played a key role in the building and maintaining of hospitals. Many hospitals were built and maintained by bishops in their respective prefectures. Hospitals were usually built near or around churches, and great importance was laid on the idea of healing through salvation. When medicine failed, doctors would ask their patients to pray. This often involved icons of Cosmas and Damien, patron saints of medicine and doctors.

Christianity also played a key role in propagating the idea of charity. Medicine was made, according to Oregon State University historian, Gary Ferngren (professor of ancient Greek and Rome history with a speciality in ancient medicine) "accessible to all and... simple".

3.2.4 See also

- Paul of Aegina
- Medical Compendium in Seven Books
- Islamic medicine
- Vienna Dioscurides
- Medieval medicine
- History of medicine

3.2.5 References

- John Scarborough, ed., *Symposium on Byzantine Medicine, Dumbarton Oaks Papers* **38** (1985) ISBN 0-88402-139-4 (not seen)
- Owsei Temkin, "Byzantine Medicine: Tradition and Empiricism", *Dumbarton Oaks Papers* **16**:97-115 (1962) at JSTOR

3.2.6 External links

- Vienna Dioscuride
- Deno Geanakoplos
- Paul of Aegina: Epitome - On The Fracture of the Thigh and Nose

3.3 Cupping therapy

Cupping therapy is an ancient form of alternative medicine in which a local suction is created on the skin; practitioners believe this mobilizes blood flow in order to promote healing.[1] Suction is created using heat (fire) or mechanical devices (hand or electrical pumps). [2]

3.3.1 Description

Through either heat or suction, the skin is gently drawn upwards by creating a vacuum in a cup over the target area of the skin. The cup stays in place for five to fifteen minutes. It is believed by some to help treat pain, deep scar tissues in the muscles and connective tissue, muscle knots, and swelling.

3.3.2 History

There is reason to believe the practice dates from as early as 3000 BC. The Ebers Papyrus, written c. 1550 BC and one of the oldest medical textbooks in the world, describes the Egyptians' use of cupping. Archaeologists have found evidence in China of cupping dating back to 1000 BC. In ancient Greece, Hippocrates (c. 400 BC) used cupping for internal disease and structural problems. This method in multiple forms spread into medicine throughout Asian and European civilizations. In 1465, cupping was recommended Serefeddin Sabuncuoglu, a Turkish surgeon, and called it mihceme.[3]

3.3.3 Methods

Broadly speaking there are two types of cupping: dry cupping and bleeding or wet cupping (controlled bleeding) with wet cupping being more common. The British Cupping Society (BCS), an organisation promoting the practice, teaches both. As a general rule, wet cupping provides a more "curative-treatment approach" to patient management whereas dry cupping appeals more to a "therapeutic and relaxation approach". Preference varies with practitioners and cultures.

Dry cupping

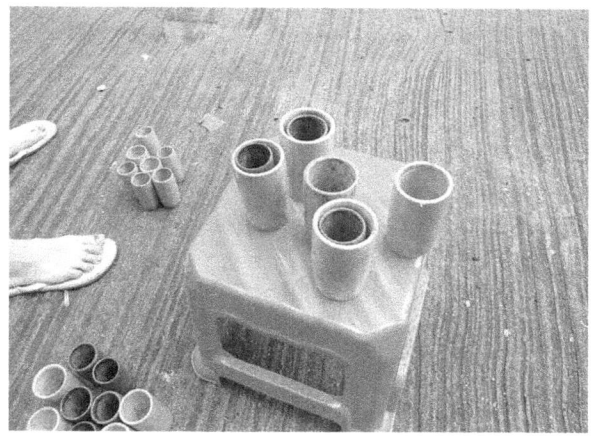

Bamboo cups

The cupping procedure commonly involves creating a small area of low air pressure next to the skin. However, there is variety in the tools used, the method of creating the low pressure, and the procedures followed during the treatment.[4]

The cups can be various shapes including balls or bells, and may range in size from 1 to 3 inches (25 to 76 mm) across the opening. Plastic and glass are the most common materials used today, replacing the horn, pottery, bronze and bamboo cups used in earlier times. The low air pressure required may be created by heating the cup or the air inside it with an open flame or a bath in hot scented oils, then placing it against the skin. As the air inside the cup cools, it contracts and draws the skin slightly inside. More recently, vacuum can be created with a mechanical suction pump acting through a valve located at the top of the cup. Rubber cups are also available that squeeze the air out and adapt to uneven or bony surfaces.

In practice, cups are normally used only on softer tissue that can form a good seal with the edge of the cup. They may be used singly or with many to cover a larger area. They may be used by themselves or placed over an acupuncture needle. Skin may be lubricated, allowing the cup to move across the skin slowly.

Depending on the specific treatment, skin marking is common after the cups are removed. This may be a simple red ring that disappears quickly, the discolouration left by the cups is normally from bruising especially if dragging the cups while suctioned from one place to another to break down muscle fiber. Usually treatments are not painful.

Fire cupping

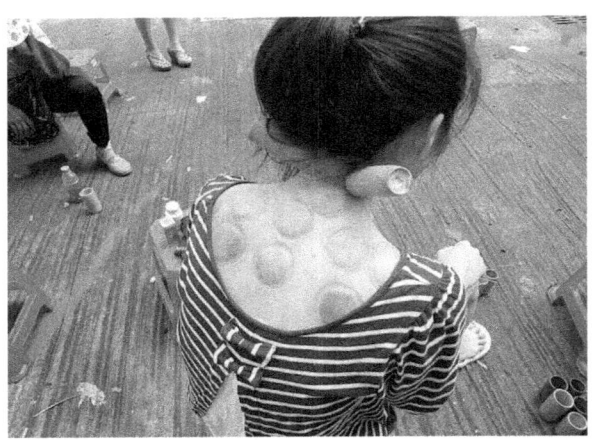

A woman receiving fire cupping at a roadside business in Haikou, Hainan, China.

Fire cupping involves soaking a cotton ball in 70% alcohol. The cotton is then clamped by a pair of forceps and lit via match or lighter. The flaming cotton ball is then, in one fluid motion, placed into the cup, quickly removed, and the cup is placed on the skin. By adding fire to the inside of the cup, oxygen is removed (which is replaced with an equal volume of carbon dioxide) and a small amount of suction is created by the air cooling down again and contracting. Massage oil may be applied to create a better seal as well as allow the

cups to glide over muscle groups (e.g. trapezius, erectors, latisimus dorsi, etc.) in an act called "moving cupping". Dark circles may appear where the cups were placed due to rupture of the capillaries just under the skin, but are not the same as a bruise caused by blunt-force trauma.

Wet cupping (Al-Hijamah or medicinal bleeding)
Further information: Hijama

While the history of wet cupping may date back thousands of years, the first documented uses are found in the teachings of the Islamic prophet Muhammad.[5] According to Muhammad al-Bukhari, Muslim ibn al-Hajjaj Nishapuri and Ahmad ibn Hanbal, Muhammad approved of the Hijama (cupping) treatment.[6]

A number of hadith support its recommendation and use by Muhammad. As a result, the practice of cupping therapy has survived in Muslim countries. Today, wet cupping is a popular remedy practiced in many parts of the Muslim world .[7]

Alternatively, mild suction is created using a cup and a pump (or heat suction) on the selected area and left for about three minutes. The cup is then removed and small superficial skin incisions are made using a cupping scalpel. A second suction is used to carefully draw out a small quantity of blood. The procedure was piloted and developed by Ullah et al 2005 and has been endorsed by the British Cupping Society[1] which aims to promote, protect and develop professional standards in cupping therapy.

In Finland, wet cupping has been done at least since the 15th century, and it is done traditionally in saunas. The cupping cups were made of cattle horns with a valve mechanism in it to create an partial vacuum by sucking the air out. Cupping is still used in Finland as an alternative medicine.

3.3.4 Traditional Chinese medicine cupping

According to traditional Chinese medicine (TCM) cupping is a method of creating a vacuum on the patient's skin to dispel stagnation — stagnant blood and lymph, thereby improving qi flow — to treat respiratory diseases such as the common cold, pneumonia and bronchitis. Cupping also is used on back, neck, shoulder and other musculoskeletal conditions. Its advocates say it has other applications, as well.[8] Cupping is not advised over skin ulcers or to the abdominal or sacral regions of pregnant women.[9]

3.3.5 Limited bruising cupping

New silicone therapy cups are claimed to alleviate bruising associated with traditional cupping. The cups are easier to use and are pliable, unlike glass or plastic, allowing for home use. Due to the lack of bruising and overall comfort, silicone cups are mainly smaller in size and used for facial cupping. Hydration before and after the therapy and general massage can also help reduce the bruising from cupping.

3.3.6 Practice

Cupping is claimed to treat a broad range of medical conditions such as blood disorders (anaemia, haemophilia), rheumatic diseases (arthritic joint and muscular conditions), fertility and gynaecological disorders, and skin problems (eczema, acne), and is claimed by proponents to help general physical and psychological well-being.

There is a description of cupping in George Orwell's essay "How the Poor Die", where he was surprised to find it practiced in a Paris hospital.

3.3.7 Effectiveness

As with many forms of manual therapy, the effectiveness of cupping is difficult to determine as it virtually impossible to construct a double blind or placebo-controlled clinical trial. Developing a "sham" manual therapy for cupping would be difficult and it would be impossible to blind the therapist.

In their 2008 book *Trick or Treatment*, Simon Singh and Edzard Ernst write that no evidence exists of any beneficial effects of cupping for any medical condition.[10]

Cupping is widely used as an alternative treatment for cancer. However, the American Cancer Society notes that "available scientific evidence does not support claims that cupping has any health benefits" and also that the treatment carries a small risk of burns.[2]

A 2012 review of the evidence in an article published in PLOS ONE said that studies appeared to show that cupping therapy was effective for treating a number of conditions, but that "nearly all included trials were evaluated as high risk of bias" – better designed studies would be needed in order to reach definitive conclusions.[11]

Very few scientific studies have been conducted on the validity of cupping as an alternative medical practice. In fact, a significant amount of studies either do not support cupping practices or are unable to reach a conclusion concerning its effectiveness.

Traditional Persian medicine in Iran takes advantage of wet cupping practices, for the belief that cupping with scarification may eliminate the scar tissue, and cupping without scarification would cleanse the body through the organs (Nimrouzi et al., 2014).[12] Research suggests that this practice is indeed harmful, especially to thin or obese patients. It may be noted that individuals of profound interest in the practice are religious and seek purification. According to Jack Raso (1997),[13] cupping results in capillary expansion, excessive fluid accumulation in tissues, and the rupture of blood vessels. Although bruising caused by this practice is common, minor, and temporary, continuation may cause burns of the skin. Individuals have been performing the action for over 3,000 years, it is still yet to be scientifically proven. The practice is performed unsupervised, without any medical background, and often indicates more risks than obvious benefits.

In a recent controlled study by Cho and colleagues (2014),[14] traditional East-Asian medical practices were evaluated in terms of effectiveness against lower back pain. Cupping was evaluated by the current Clinical Practice Guidelines (CPGs) and with evidence from current systematic reviews and meta-analyses. They found that out of thirteen CPGs, only one recommended cupping. The researchers therefore weakly recommended cupping for both (sub) acute and chronic lower back pain. Due to a belief in its benefits stemming from traditional uses, it may be that cupping induces a placebo effect rather than any direct medical benefits.

3.3.8 See also

- Gua Sha
- Hijama
- List of ineffective cancer treatments
- Moxibustion

3.3.9 References

[1] "British Cupping Society". Retrieved 2008.

[2] "Cupping". American Cancer Society. November 2008. Archived from the original on 6 April 2015. Retrieved 4 October 2013.

[3] Kaya SO, Karatepe M, Tok T, Onem G, Dursunoglu N, Goksin, I (September 2009). "Were pneumothorax and its management known in 15th-century anatolia?". *Texas Heart Institute Journal* **36** (2): 152–153. PMC 2676596. PMID 19436812.

[4] Cui Jin and Zhang Guangqi, "A survey of thirty years' clinical application of cupping", Journal of Traditional Chinese Medicine 1989; 9(3): 151–154

[5] Andrew Rippin and Jan Knappert, *Textual Sources for the Study of Islam,* Manchester: Manchester University Press, 1986; Chicago: University of Chicago Press, 1990. 78.

[6] Sunan Abu Dawood, 11:2097, 28:3848, Sahih Muslim, 26:5467, 10:3830

[7] Observations of the popularity and religious significance of blood-cupping (al-ḥijāma) as an Islamic medicine, Ahmed El-Wakil, *Contemporary Islamic Studies,* Vol. 2011, 2

[8] State Administration of Traditional Chinese Medicine and Pharmacy, *Advanced Textbook on Traditional Chinese Medicine and Pharmacology,* Volume IV, 1997 New World Press, Beijing

[9] Chinese Acupuncture and Moxibustion (Revised Edition), Xingnong, Foreign Languages Press, Beijing, China, 1987, p370.

[10] Singh, Simon; Ernst, Edzard (2008). *Trick or Treatment.* Transworld Publishers. p. 368. ISBN 9780552157629.

[11] Cao, Huijuan; Li, Xun; Liu, Jianping (2012). "An updated review of the efficacy of cupping therapy". *PLoS ONE* **7** (2): e31793. doi:10.1371/journal.pone.0031793. PMC 3289625. PMID 22389674.

[12] http://chp.sagepub.com.qe2a-proxy.mun.ca/content/19/2/128.full.pdf+html

[13] http://skepdic.com/cupping.html

[14] http://web.a.ebscohost.com.qe2a-proxy.mun.ca/ehost/pdfviewer/pdfviewer?sid=885e36e3-8b04-4342-a94f-74ee840166fe%40sessionmgr4003&vid=16&hid=4106

3.3.10 External links

- Cupping Directory

- The efficacy of wet-cupping in the treatment of tension and migraine headache.

- Traditional Cupping Film

- British Cupping Society website

- Cupping online journal

- Cupping Resource

3.4 Dodecapharmacum

A **dodecapharmacum** is a medicine of twelve ingredients.[1]

The best known was the **Apostles' Ointment** (Latin: Apostolorum unguentum), or **Ointment of Venus** (Latin: unguentum Veneris) which was an ointment attributed to Avicenna (d.1037) made of twelve ingredients. The ingredients were turpentine, wax, gum ammoniac, birthwort roots, olibanum, bdellium, myrrh and galbanum, opoponax, verdigris, litharge, plus olive oil, and vinegar.[2][3]

Avicenna describes the ingredients and proportions of such a recipe in Qanun V.1.11. Some later writers have questioned whether the title of the recipe "Ointment of the Apostles," or "Ointment of Venus" were used by Avicenna himself,[4] however when an Arabic version of the Canon of Medicine (القانون في الطب) was first printed in 1593 in Rome, recipe no. 442 (Arabic ٤٤٢) was entitled "ointment of the Apostles" (Arabic: مرهم الرسل *marham ur rusul*).[5] The name "Ointment of the Apostles" for the 12-ingredient recipe appears in the works of the Dominican priest Teodorico Borgognoni (1267)[6] and the *Inventarium sive chirugia magna* of Guy de Chauliac (1330s).[7] Renaissance pharmacy texts such as the *Antidotarium Romanum* (Rome, 1590) also include the recipe as *Unguentem Apostolorum*.[8] The Arabic equivalent of the Latin *Unguentum Apostolorum* is found in later Arabic medical texts such as the translations into Arabic of the Nestorian Christian physician David of Antioch (d.1596).[9][10][11][12]

Naming of the ointment of the Apostles as ointment of Venus occurs in the works of Jehan Yperman (c.1260-c.1330). [13] However many remedies were called "..of Venus" and also widely known in antiquity was an eye-salve called "the plaster of Isis" distinct from later "Ointment of Venus."[14]

Mirza Ghulam Ahmad (Urdu 1899) claimed that this ointment was known as the "Ointment of Jesus" (Arabic: مرهم عيسى marham-i-Isa) and had helped Jesus recover from the wounds of crucifixion, in support of his claim that Jesus did not die upon the Cross and was saved. Mirza Ghulam Ahmad claimed that he was the Promised Messiah and Mahdi.[15]

3.4.1 References

[1] Robley Dunglison *Medical Lexicon* 1857 "An ancient name given to all medicines which consisted of 12 ingredients"

[2] *The London encyclopaedia: or Universal dictionary of science, art, ...* Volume 2 1829 - Page 507 "It was invented by Avicenna, and is also called unguentum veneris. The ingredients are turpentine, wax, gum ammoniac, birthwort roots, olibanum, bdellium, myrrh and galbanum, opoponax, verdigris, litharge, oil of olives, and vinegar."

[3] Denis Diderot, Benard Encyclopédie ou Dictionnaire raisonné des sciences, des arts et ... 1778 - Page 47 "L'onguent des apôtres, en Pharmacie, est une espece d'onguent qui déterge ou netoie : il est composé de douze

drogues; c'est la raison pourquoi il est nommé l'onguent des apôtres. Voyez ONGUENT. Avicenne en fut l'inventeur."

[4] Société de médecine de Gand - 1854 "Il est peu probable que l'Arabe Avicenne ait appelé cet onguent l'onguent de Vénus ou des douze apôtres. Cet onguent sera introduit dans la plaie.."

[5] Rome printed edition 1593 online at American Embassy of Beirut entry No.442 at head of page

[6] The surgery of Theodoric: ca. A.D. 1267 - Volume 2 - Page 15 Teodorico (dei Borgognoni) - 1960 "Avicenna says, "And the root of hart's tongue has already been tested, for when a fistula is filled with this, it heals it. ... There are also: The ointment of Venus, which is called the ointment of the twelve apostles, which Avicenna applies. Also"

[7] fr:Guy de Chauliac (1298-1368) *Inventarium sive chirugia magna* Volume 14,Part 2 ed. M. Michael Rogers McVaugh - 1997 - Page 177 "Avicenna describes unguentum apostolorum et est apostolicon in Canon V.1. 11 (533va), "rectificans cum facilitate fistulas difficiles": "Rx terebentine cere albe et resine omnium ana dr. 14; oppoponaci et floris eris amborum ana 2 ammoniaci pon. dr. 14; aristo. longe et thuris masculi amborum ana dr. 6.; myrrhe et galbani amborum ana dr. 4; bdellii pon. dr. 6; lithargyrii pond. dr. 9.; infundatur bdellium in aceto vini et decoquatur in estate cum duabus lib. olei et in hyeme cum lib. 3." Dino, Compilatio, [154]va, explains "dicitur unguentum apostolorum quia in eo sunt 12 medicine"; his ingredients are those of the Canon except that he leaves out terebentina — something obviously had to be omitted if he was to end with twelve rather than thirteen."

[8] *Antidotarium Romanum: seu modus componendi medicamenta* 1590 p93 "Recipe terebentinae.." p94 "Resinae. Ammoniaci an drach quatordecim."

[9] Dawud al-Antaki, Tadhkirat uli al-albab wa-l-jami'li-lil-ajab al-ujjab. Cairo, reprint 1935.

[10] al-'Attar Haruni *Minhaj al-dukkan wa-dustur al-a'yan* 1992
"مرهم الرسل، وهو مرهم لعفنة ا . الخبيبيثة المزمنة"
ثا٢١ يدمل الجراحا٠١لمتطاولة، ويني بالعيراني الرسل.
ثلبقعرنأيلبئئئكئرما يؤخذ شمع أبيض البواسير.
جنندرسم اهم د ستة ٢ اهم د ونيإ ويك دل الخنازير بقايا ويحلل
مراهد ٩. ٠٠٠. ا ٠ركندو طويل دناوند وزراوند همنيتوار ".

[11] Abu Bakr ibn Badr al-Din Baytar, 'Abd al-Raḥmān Ibrīq *Kamil al-sanaàtayn fi al-baytarah wa-al-zardaqah* 1993 "...
شاء المتم تعالى ج صفة مرهم الرسل النافع لجميع
الجراحات ويدمل الجراحات ؛ يؤخذ شمع، ومرتك، وراتينج
بالسوية، وجاوشير، وقنة، وهر، وزنجار، من كل واحد رع جزء
لمستعمل والزيت بالذياب ويذاب إحني عيني الجميع يدق ٠١صضة
"... مرهم الداخلون النافع لجميع الأورام في الاعضاء"

[12] Louis Robert Effler *My scrapbook of medicine: a series of squibs in prose and verse* 1937 Page 36 "We must not confuse truly scientific attempts at medicine-making with such pseudo-scientific efforts as "the ointment of the twelve apostles." This, as may be supposed, contained twelve ingredients and ranked with such of our modern nostrums as "Father John's Remedy" and others. Such a religious aroma has been well calculated to snare the unwary from the earliest times to the present."

[13] Jan Yperman, Leonard D. Rosenman *The surgery of Master Jehan Yperman (1260?−1330?)* 2002 Page 131 "Afterwards, dress the wound with lint from an old linen cloth coated with the ointment of the Twelve Apostles, which Avicenna first made and named it unguentum veneris duodecim apostolorum." The ointment is useful in fistulas (ie chronic) ..."

[14] The American Encyclopedia and Dictionary of Ophthalmology (1916) cited in Jean-Paul Wayenborgh, Saiichi Mishima, C. Richard Keeler IBBO: A-K - Page 407 - 2001 "Long and widely known in antiquity was the eye-salve called "the plaster of Isis." Isis would, in fact, appear to have been, among the gods, "a general practitioner, paying especial attention to diseases of the eye."

[15] Yohanan Friedmann *The Messianic Claim of Ghulam Ahmad* in *Toward the Millennium: Messianic Expectations from the Bible to Waco* ed. Peter Schäfer, Mark R. Cohen, Brill 1998 p299-310 p306: "Jesus was therefore taken down from the cross, cured of his wounds with a special ointment known as "the ointment of Jesus" (marham-i-Isa), went to India to look for the lost tribes of Israel... Having proven to his own satisfaction that the crucifixion attempt was a failure and that Jesus died a natural death, Ghulam Ahmad was now ready to address the issue of his second coming. ... This person is Ghulam Ahmad himself, whom God transformed into Jesus and sent to silence the Christians,..."

3.5 Exorcism in Islam

Exorcism in Islam is called *ruqya*. It is used to repair the damage caused by *sihr* or witchcraft. Exorcisms today are part of a wider body of contemporary Islamic alternative medicine called **al-Tibb al-Nabawi** (Medicine of the Prophet).[1]

3.5.1 Islamic religious context

Further information: Devil and Jinn

Muslims believe in the concept of a malevolent Devil. Belief in Jinns, or supernatural beings, is also widespread in the Islamic world.[2][3][68[4]:193:34]

A related belief is that every person is assigned one's own special jinnī, also called a *qarīn* (also called a hamzaad in India & Pakistan), of the jinn that whisper to people's souls and tell them to submit to evil desires.[5][6][7] The notion of a *qarīn* is not universally accepted amongst all Muslims,

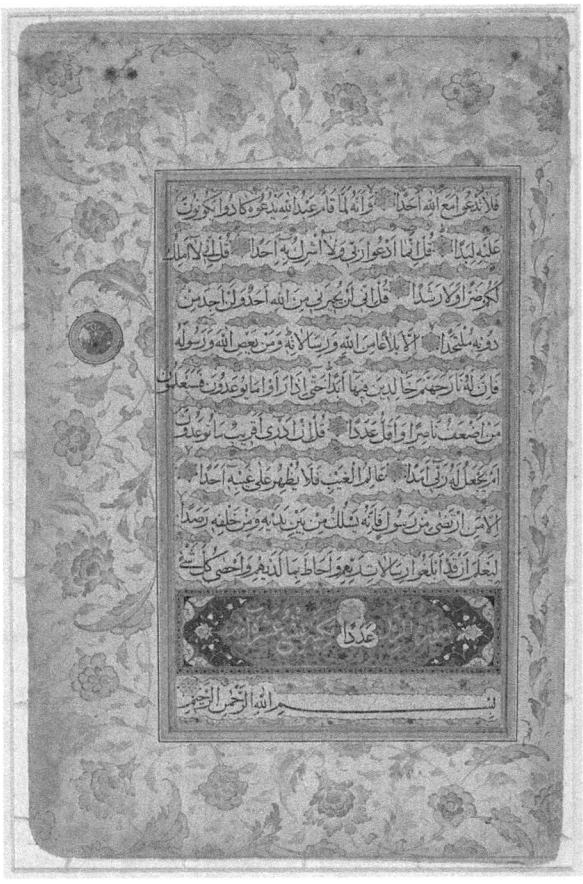

The 72nd chapter of the Qur'an entitled al-Jinn (the Spirits), as well as the heading and introductory bismillah of the next chapter entitled al-Muzzammil (The Enshrouded One).

but it is generally accepted that Šayṭān whispers in human minds, and he is assigned to each human being.[8]

3.5.2 Procedure

Islamic exorcisms consist of the treated person lying down, while a white-gloved therapist places a hand on a patient's head while chanting verses from the Quran.[1] The drinking of holy water may also take place.[9]

Specific verses from the Quran are recited, which glorify God (e.g. The Throne Verse (Arabic: آية الكرسي *Ayatul Kursi*), and invoke God's help. In some cases, the *adhan*/"ah-zan" (the call for daily prayers) is also read, as this has the effect of repelling non-angelic unseen beings or the *jinn*.

The Islamic prophet Muhammad taught his followers to read the last three *suras* from the Quran, Surat al-Ikhlas (The Fidelity), Surat al-Falaq (The Dawn) and Surat al-Nas (Mankind).

(e.g. The Throne Verse (Arabic: آية الكرسي *Ayatul Kursi*) :-

3.5.3 Popularity of Islamic alternative medicine

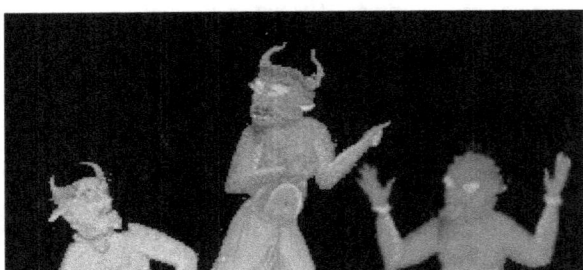

Ali and the Jinn, *Golestan Palace, Iran, 1568.*

The trend in *al-Tibb al-Nabawi* treatments, cosmetics and toiletries is often associated with fundamentalists who charge that Western, chemically laced prescriptions aim to poison Muslims or defile them with insulin and other medicines made from pigs.[1] Members of terrorist groups have been involved in Islamic remedies as healers and sellers, while some clinics are used as recruiting grounds for Islamist causes.[1]

"Islamic medicine carries a cachet that, by taking it, you are reinforcing your faith – and the profits go to Muslims," says Sidney Jones, an expert on Islam in Southeast Asia with the International Crisis Group.[1]

3.5.4 Court Cases

In 2012, six people sat trial in a Belgium court in connection with the 2004 murder of a young Muslim woman in a deadly act of exorcism.[9] Her body was found covered with bruises, and her lungs filled with water.[9]

The detainees in the case include two self-appointed exorcists, the victim's husband and three female members of a radical Muslim group.[9] Her husband later admitted to investigators that his wife was subjected month-long sessions of exorcism to evict from her body the demons that "prevented her from becoming pregnant."[9]

During this period, the young woman had swallowed liters of holy water, according to Belgian media reports. She was fed two spoons of yogurt every day and always had earphones playing verses from the Quran.[9] In order to evict the demons, the exorcists reportedly put their fingers down the woman's throat, forced her into bathing in hot water and beat her with a stick.[9]

Also, on October 18th 2012, a British court convicted[10]

three men of assault and causing actual bodily harm after they had beaten a female family member they believed showed signs of demonic possession. She was beaten for almost eight hours on January 7th, 2011. A fourth suspect, remains at large.

3.5.5 See also

- Devil

- Jinn

3.5.6 References

[1] Hallowell, Billy (26 September 2011). "Some Asian Muslims Giving Up Western Meds for Islamic Exorcisms & Treatments". *TheBlaze*.

[2] Quran 51:56–56

[3] al-Ṭabarī, Muḥammad ibn Ayyūb. *Tuḥfat al-gharāʼib* I.

[4] Rāzī, =Abū al-Futūḥ. *Tafsīr-e rawḥ al-jenān va rūḥ al-janān*.

[5] Quran 72:1–2

[6] Quran 15:18–18

[7] *Sahih Muslim*, No. 2714

[8] *Is it permissible to pray that my qareen becomes Muslim*

[9] Staff (14 May 2012). "Belgium court charges six people in deadly exorcism of Muslim woman". *Al Arabiya*.

[10] Staff Reporter (22 October 2012). "Jail for brutal attack on defenceless mother". *East End Life*.

3.5.7 External links

Ruqyah treatment

3.6 Hijama

Hijama (Arabic: حجامة lit. "sucking") is the Arabic traditional medicine for wet cupping, where blood is drawn by vacuum from a small skin incision for therapeutic purposes.[1] It is reported that the Islamic prophet Muhammad said, "Indeed the best of remedies you have is hijama, and if there was something excellent to be used as a remedy then it is hijama."[2]

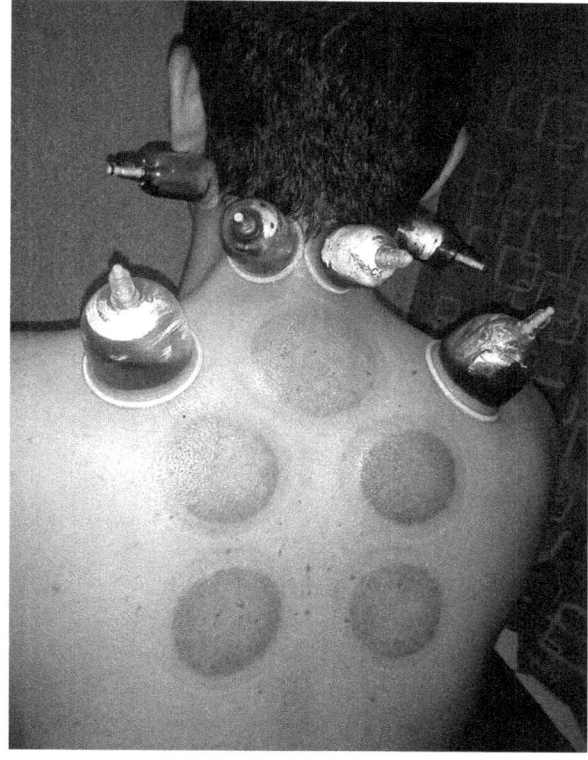

Hijama therapy.

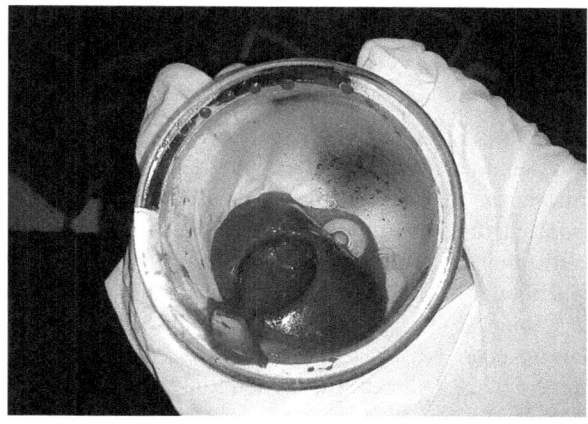

Clotted blood after being drawn by wet cupping.

3.6.1 Procedure

Hijama can be performed almost anywhere on the body, often at the site of an ache or pain in order to ease or alleviate it. A more conservative approach[3] warns against over use of cupping and suggests only that six optimal points on the body are all that is required to "clean" the entire cardiovascular system. The location is first shaved, if necessary, to ensure a tight seal with the cup. The mouth of a cup (metal, glass and plastic cups are generally used, although traditionally horns were used) is placed on the skin at the site chosen for hijama. Then a tight seal is created. The traditional method is to burn a small piece of paper or cotton inside the vessel, so that the mouth of the cup clings to the skin. Some practitioners now use a machine instead of the manual cups. Some practitioners still strictly adhere to the Prophetic method with the use of fire, both for sterility and the benefits or properties from the element of fire itself that may be present. The cup is left to cling to the skin for a few minutes, then it is lifted off and several very small incisions are made in the skin. The cup is then put back as it was before until the flow of blood subsides. Hijama is considered a form of energy medicine because it has been claimed to unclog the meridians in the body, and is viewed by some practitioners as a cure that can alleviate black magic and possession.[4]

3.6.2 Scientific Studies

In March 2011 three systematic reviews were analyzed for the effectiveness of wet and dry cupping in which two out of three showed some evidence for effectiveness of cupping for pain. Favorable effects were shown when wet cupping was combined with adjuvant conventional treatments. However, one of the three reviews showed little effectivess for cupping for stroke rehabilitation. Few randomized control trials have been done to examine the effectiveness of cupping and many studies published are of low quality or have many limitations.[5]

A study by Ahmed and colleagues was carried out in order to evaluate the efficiency of cupping [hijama] therapy in management of rheumatoid arthritis. To sum up they concluded cupping [hijama] combined with conventional medical therapy has several advantages. It significantly reduces the laboratory markers of disease activity and it modulates the immune cellular conditions particularly of innate immune response NK cell % and adaptive cellular immune response SIL-20 (Ahmed, Madbouly, Maklad $ Abu-Shady, 2005)[6]

Using a pre-post research design, 70 patients with chronic tension or migraine headache were treated with wet-cupping. Three primary outcome measures were considered at the baseline and 3 months following treatment: headache severity, days of headache per month, and use of medication. Results suggest that, compared to the baseline, mean headache severity decreased by 66% following wet-cupping treatment. Treated patients also experienced the equivalent of 12.6 fewer days of headache per month. We conclude that wet-cupping leads to clinical relevant benefits for primary care patients with headache. Possible mechanisms of wet-cupping's efficacy, as well as directions for future research are discussed.[7]

There is some evidence that wet-cupping is effective in the treatment of nonspecific low back pain.[8] Studies have also shown some evidence that it may be effective in the treatment of post-herpetic neuralgia.[9] For the treatment of cancer, there is no scientific evidence to suggest that hijama confers any health benefits.[10]

3.6.3 Bloodletting Comparison

While often used interchangeably, hijama and bloodletting are not similar techniques. Bloodletting opens veins and bleeds patients, whereas hijama draws blood to a specific location with suction and extracts it by perforating the skin. "A study by Bilal and colleagues was aimed by comparing and analyzing the difference between the compositions of blood samples, obtained through cupping (hijama) technique versus blood drawn intravenously. There was a significant change in almost all parameters tested as compared to the venous blood samples to scientifically evaluate the efficacy of the techniques used in cupping (hijama) i.e. suction and removal of blood." (Bilal, ALam Khan, Ahmed & Afroz, 2011)[11]

3.6.4 Practitioners

Cupping [hijama] remained a constant in professional medical treatment throughout Europe. It was practiced by such famous physicians as Galen (131-200AD), Paracelsus (1493-1541) and Ambroise Pare (1509–90). Cupping [hijama] was also practiced by other practitioners including barbers, surgeons and bath house attendants. (Chirali, 1999)

3.6.5 Safety

Cupping has few major side effects aside from the pain of skin cuts. One potentially serious risk is infection. Other possible minor side effects that may occur is feeling of slight light headedness post therapy, this is similar to the sensation one feels after having blood taken when donating blood. Cupping [hijama] encourages blood flow to the cupped region (hyperemia), one may therefore feel warmer and hotter as a result of vasodilatation taking place and slight sweating may occur. Pregnant women or menstruating women, cancer (metastatic) patients and patients with bone fractures or muscle spasms are also believed to be contra-indicated. Some practitioners suggest that a low risk of blood clotting is possible and therefore walking and staying awake after a procedure is advisable.[12]

3.6.6 See also

- Bloodletting
- Ijaza
- Fire cupping
- Medicine in medieval Islam
- Blood donation
- Hematology
- History of medicine

3.6.7 References

[1] Traditional Medicine Among Gulf Arabs Part II - Blood Letting, Albinali, H. A. Hâyar, *Heart Views*, Volume 5, No.2, June–August 2004

[2] Al Jauziyah & Abdullah, 2003

[3] Cupping, Hijama, Buhwang . . .

[4] Observations of the popularity and religious significance of blood-cupping (al-ḥijāma) as an Islamic medicine, Ahmed El-Wakil, *Contemporary Islamic Studies*, Vol. 2011, 2

[5] FACT, Focus on Alternative and Complementary Therapies, Abdullah AlBedah,Mohamed Khalil, Ahmed Elolemy, Ibrahim Elsubai, Asim Khalil, *Hijama (cupping): a review of the evidence*, Volume 16, Issue 1, pages 12–16, March 2011

[6] FACT, Focus on Alternative and Complementary Therapies, Abdullah AlBedah,Mohamed Khalil, Ahmed Elolemy, Ibrahim Elsubai, Asim Khalil, *Hijama (cupping): a review of the evidence*, Volume 16, Issue 1, pages 12–16, March 2011

[7] http://www.worldscientific.com/doi/abs/10.1142/S0192415X08005564

[8] "The effectiveness of wet-cupping for nonspecific low back pain in Iran: a randomized controlled trial.". *Complement Ther Med* **17** (1): 9–15. Jan 2009. doi:10.1016/j.ctim.2008.05.003. PMID 19114223.

[9] http://www.ncbi.nlm.nih.gov/pmc/articles/PMC3151529/

[10] http://www.cancer.org/Treatment/TreatmentsandSideEffects/ComplementaryandAlternativeMedicine/HerbsVitaminsandMinerals/cupping

[11] Evaluation of the Effects of Traditional Cupping [Hijama] on the Biochemical, Hematological and Immunological Factors of Human Venous Blood. Muahmmad Reza, et al., Shahed University, Faculty of Medicine, Islamic Republic of Iran, *A Compendium of Essays on Alternative Therapy*, Bilal, et al. Partial Evaluation of Techniques Used in Cupping [hijama] [original] Journal of Basic and Applied Science, 7, 65-68

[12] FACT, Focus on Alternative and Complementary Therapies, Abdullah AlBedah,Mohamed Khalil, Ahmed Elolemy, Ibrahim Elsubai, Asim Khalil, *Hijama (cupping): a review of the evidence*, Volume 16, Issue 1, page 5, March 2011

3.6.8 Further reading

- Mahdavi, M. (2011). "Evaluation of the Effects of Traditional Cupping on the Biochemical, Hematological and Immunological Factors of Human Venous Blood" (PDF). *A Compendium of Essays on Alternative Therapy*. Retrieved 17 March 2013.

3.7 Medicine in the medieval Islamic world

This article is about Historic practice of "Rational medicine". For Islam in medicine, see Prophetic medicine. For the contemporary practice, see Unani.

In the history of medicine, **Islamic medicine**, **Ara-**

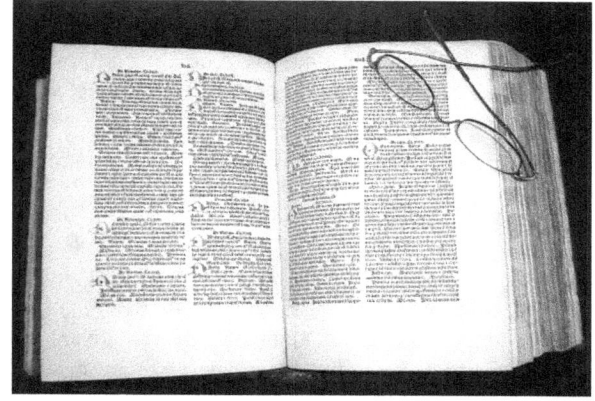

A Latin copy of the Canon of Medicine, dated 1484, located at the P.I. Nixon Medical Historical Library of The University of Texas Health Science Center at San Antonio.

bic medicine, **Greco-Arabic** and **Greco-Islamic** refer to medicine developed in the Islamic Golden Age, and written in Arabic, the *lingua franca* of Islamic civilization. The emergence of Islamic medicine came about through the interactions of the indigenous Arab tradition with foreign influences.[1] Translation of earlier texts was a fundamental building block in the formation of Islamic medicine and the tradition that has been passed down.[1]

Latin translations of Arabic medical works had a significant influence on the development of medicine in the high Middle Ages and early Renaissance, as did Arabic texts which translated the medical works of earlier cultures.[2]

The mind-body connection is inherent to Islamic medicine, whose foundations are Imaan (faith) and Tawakkul (trust). According to the Islamic prophet, Muhammad: "There is no disease that Allah has created, except that He also has created its remedy." (Bukhari).[3] Indeed, this lay the foundations for early medical science, for "the Prophet not only instructed sick people to take medicine, but he himself invited expert physicians for this purpose".[4] Around the ninth century, the Islamic medical community began to develop and utilize a system of medicine based on scientific analysis.[5] The importance of the health sciences to society was emphasized, and the early Muslim medical community strived to find ways to care for the health of the human body. Medieval Islam developed hospitals, expanded the practice of surgery. Important medical thinkers and physicians of this time were Al-Razi (Rhazes) and Ibn Sina (Avicenna). Their knowledge on medicine was recorded in books that were influential in medical schools throughout Muslim world and Europe, and Ibn Sina in particular (under his Latinized name Avicenna) was also influential on the physicians of later medieval Europe. Throughout the medieval Islamic world, medicine was included under the umbrella of natural philosophy, due to the continued influence of the Hippocratic Corpus and the ideas of Aristotle and Galen. The Hippocratic Corpus was a collection of medical treatises attributed to the famous Greek physician Hippocrates of Cos (although it was actually composed by different generations of authors). The Corpus included a number of treatises which greatly influenced medieval Islamic medical literature.

3.7.1 Terminology

Some consider the label "Arab-Islamic" as historically inaccurate, arguing it does not appreciate the rich diversity of scholars who contributed to Islamic science, many of whom were neither Arab nor Muslim.[6][7]

3.7.2 Overview

Medicine was a central part of medieval Islamic culture. Responding to circumstances of time and place, Islamic physicians and scholars developed a large and complex medical literature exploring, analyzing, and synthesizing the theory and practice of medicine.[8] Islamic medicine was initially built on tradition, chiefly the theoretical and practical knowledge developed in Arabia and was known at Muhammad's time, ancient Hellenistic medicine such

as Unani, ancient Indian medicine such as Ayurveda, and the ancient Iranian Medicine of the Academy of Gundishapur. The works of ancient Greek and Roman physicians Hippocrates,[9] Galen and Dioscorides[9] also had a lasting impact on Islamic medicine.[10] Ophthalmology has been described as the most successful branch of medicine researched at the time, with the works of Ibn Al-Haitham remaining an authority in the field until early modern times.[11]

3.7.3 Medical ethics

The earliest surviving Arabic work on medical ethics is Ishaq ibn 'Ali al-Ruhawi's Adab al-Tabib ("Practical Ethics of the Physician" or "Practical Medical Deontology") and was based on the works of Hippocrates and Galen.[7] Al-Ruhawi regarded physicians as "guardians of souls and bodies", and wrote twenty chapters on various topics related to medical ethics.[12]

Encyclopedias

The first encyclopedia of medicine in Arabic language[13] was by Persian scientist Ali ibn Sahl Rabban al-Tabari's Firdous al-Hikmah ("Paradise of Wisdom"), written in seven parts, c. 860. Al-Tabari, a pioneer in the field of child development, emphasized strong ties between psychology and medicine, and the need for psychotherapy and counseling in the therapeutic treatment of patients. His encyclopedia also discussed the influence of Sushruta and Chanakya on medicine, including psychotherapy.[14]

3.7.4 Major contributors to Muslim medicine

> The art of healing was dead, Galen revived it;
> it was scattered and dis-arrayed, Razi re-arranged
> and re-aligned it; it was incomplete, Ibn Sinna
> perfected it.[15]

Ali ibn Mousa al-Ridha

Ali ibn Mousa al-Ridha, the eighth Imam of shia (765-818), was at the top of the scientists of his time in medical science, and his treatise in medicine is regarded as most precious Islamic literature in the science of medicine. It has been called the Golden Dissertation.[16][17]

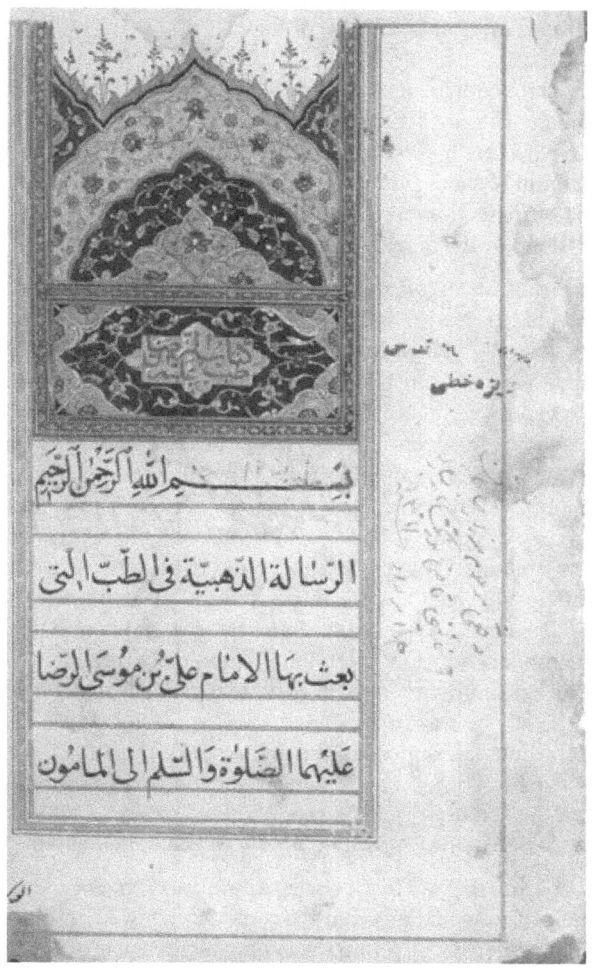

A manuscript of Al-Risalah al-Dhahabiah by Ali al-Ridha, the eighth Imam of Shia Muslims. The text says:"Golden dissertation in medicine which is sent by Imam Ali ibn Musa al-Ridha, peace be upon him, to al-Ma'mun.

Ali ibn al-'Abbas al-Majusi

'Ali ibn al-'Abbas al-Majusi (died 982-994), also known as Haly Abbas, was famous for the Kitab al-Maliki or *Complete Book of the Medical Art*, his textbook on medicine.[18]

Muhammad ibn Zakariya al-Razi

Zakariya Razi, commonly known as Rhazes, was a Persian physician, alchemist and chemist, philosopher, scholar, and a prominent figure in Islamic Golden Age. He was the chief surgeon in many hospitals in the cities of Rey and Baghdad, and he became an advisor to caliphs and rulers of the time.[19] Thanks to his authority and achievements in medicine, he was considered as the father of Islamic medicine, "the greatest physician of the Muslim World",[19]

as well as a respected philosopher. He believed in the existence of God and the soul but rejected prophetically revealed religion and ritualism, believing instead that anyone could use reason to understand the world.[20]

He is known for separating the "science of physic"[19] into two different aspects: physical and spiritual. The physical dealt with the "physiological diseases"[19] while the latter dealt with the spiritual self. He felt that in order to completely understand the science of the body, a doctor needed to be a master of both the physical and spiritual knowledge regarding the body.[19] Al-Razi was also interested in medical ethics, about which he wrote *Ahlaq al-Tabeeb*.[19] In *Ahlaq Al-Tabeeb* (*Medical Ethics*) al-Razi wrote about the importance of morality in medicine. He presented the first model for ethics in Islamic medicine. He felt that it was important not only for the physician to be an expert in his field, but also to be a role model. His ideas on medical ethics were divided into three concepts: the physician's responsibility to patients and to self, and also the patients' responsibility to physicians.[19]

In addition to being a famous physician, al-Razi is known for being an encyclopedic scholar,[15] compiling more than 200 works during his lifetime, half of them on medicine. He wrote the *Comprehensive Book of Medicine* in the 9th century. The *Large Comprehensive* was the most sought after of all his compositions, in which Rhazes recorded clinical cases of his own experience and provided very useful recordings of various diseases. Al-Razi was "the first of the (physicians of medieval Islam) to treat medicine in a comprehensive and encyclopedic manner, surpassing probably in voluminousness Galen himself...Rhazes is deservedly remembered as having first described small-pox and measles in an accurate manner".[21]

The *kitab-al Hawi fi al-tibb* (*The Comprehensive book of medicine, Continens Liber, The Virtuous Life*) was one of his largest works, a collection of medical notes that al-Razi made throughout his life in the form of extracts from his reading and observations from his own medical experience.[22][23][24][25] In its published form, it consists of 23 volumes. Each volume deals with specific parts or diseases of the body, although the groupings of ailments are often idiosyncratic.[22] *Al-Hawi* remained a textbook on medicine in most European universities, regarded until the seventeenth century as the most comprehensive work ever written by a medical man.[15]

al-Mansuri (*Liber almansoris, Liber medicinalis ad almansorem*) was written for "the Samanid prince Abu Salih al-Mansur ibn Ishaq, governor of Rayy."[26][27] It consists of ten books based mainly on Greek science. It was a prescribed textbook for medical students for centuries.[15] "The ninth section of the book, a detailed discussion of medical pathologies of the body from head to toe, became particularly famous and circulated in autonomous Latin translations as the *Liber Nonus*."[27][28]

Another work of al-Razi is called the *Kitab Tibb al-Muluki* (*Regius*). This book covers the treatments and cures of diseases and ailments, through dieting. It is thought to have been written for the noble class who were known for their gluttonous behavior and who frequently became ill with stomach diseases.

Other works include *A Dissertation on the causes of the Coryza which occurs in the spring when roses give forth their scent*, a tract in which al-Razi discussed why it is that one contracts coryza or common cold by smelling roses during the spring season,[15] and *Bur'al Sa'a* (*Instant cure*) in which he named medicines which instantly cured certain diseases.[15]

Abu-Ali al-Husayn ibn Abdullah ibn-Sina

Ibn Sina, more commonly known in west as Avicenna was a Persian polymath and physician of the tenth and eleventh centuries. He was known for his scientific works, but especially his writing on medicine.[29] He has been described as the "Father of Early Modern Medicine".[30] Ibn Sina is credited with many varied medical observations and discoveries, such as recognizing the potential of airborne transmission of disease, providing insight into many psychiatric conditions, recommending use of forceps in deliveries complicated by fetal distress, distinguishing central from peripheral facial paralysis and describing guinea worm infection and trigeminal neuralgia.[31] He is credited for writing two books in particular: his most famous, *al-Canon fi al Tibb* (*The Canon of Medicine*), and also *The Book of Healing*. His other works cover subjects including angelology, heart medicines, and treatment of kidney diseases.[29]

Avicenna's medicine became the representative of Islamic medicine mainly through the influence of his famous work *al-Canon fi al Tibb* (*The Canon of Medicine*).[29] The book was originally used as a textbook for instructors and students of medical sciences in the medical school of Avicenna.[29] The book is divided into 5 volumes: The first volume is a compendium of medical principles, the second is a reference for individual drugs, the third contains organ-specific diseases, the fourth discusses systemic illnesses as well as a section of preventative health measures, and the fifth contains descriptions of compound medicines.[31] The *Canon* was highly influential in medical schools and on later medical writers.[29]

3.7.5 Medical contributions from Medieval Islam

Human anatomy and physiology

It is claimed that an important advance in the knowledge of human anatomy and physiology was made by Ibn al-Nafis, but whether this was discovered via human dissection is doubtful because "al-Nafis tells us that he avoided the practice of dissection because of the shari'a and his own 'compassion' for the human body".[32][33]

The movement of blood through the human body was thought to be known due to the work of the Greek physicians.[34] However, there was the question of how the blood flowed from the right ventricle of the heart to the left ventricle, before the blood is pumped to the rest of the body.[34] According to Galen in the 2nd century, blood reached the left ventricle through invisible passages in the septum.[34] By some means, Ibn al-Nafis, a 13th-century Syrian physician, found the previous statement on blood flow from the right ventricle to the left to be false.[34] Ibn al-Nafis discovered that the ventricular septum was impenetrable, lacking any type of invisible passages, showing Galen's assumptions to be false.[34] Ibn al-Nafis discovered that the blood in the right ventricle of the heart is instead carried to the left by way of the lungs.[34] This discovery was one of the first descriptions of the pulmonary circulation,[34] although his writings on the subject were only rediscovered in the 20th century,[35] and it was William Harvey's later independent discovery which brought it to general attention.[36]

According the Ancient Greeks, vision was thought to a visual spirit emanating from the eyes that allowed an object to be perceived.[34] The 11th century Iraqi scientist Ibn al-Haytham, also known as Al-hazen in Latin, developed a radically new concept of human vision.[34] Ibn al-Haytham took a straight forward approach towards vision by explaining that the eye was an optical instrument.[34] The description on the anatomy of the eye led him to form the basis for his theory of image formation, which is explained through the refraction of light rays passing between 2 media of different densities.[34] Ibn al-Haytham developed this new theory on vision from experimental investigations.[34] In the 12th century, his *Book of Optics* was translated into Latin and continued to be studied both in the Islamic world and in Europe until the 17th century.[34]

Ahmad ibn Abi al-Ash'ath, a famous physician from Mosul, Iraq, described the physiology of the stomach in a live lion in his book *al-Quadi wa al-muqtadi*.[37] He wrote:

> "When food enters the stomach, especially
> when it is plentiful, the stomach dilates and its
> layers get stretched...onlookers thought the stomach was rather small, so I proceeded to pour jug
> after jug in its throat...the inner layer of the distended stomach became as smooth as the external
> peritoneal layer. I then cut open the stomach and

let the water out. The stomach shrank and I could see the pylorus..."[37]

Ahmad ibn Abi al-Ash'ath observed the physiology of the stomach in a live lion in 959. This description preceded William Beaumont by almost 900 years, making Ahmad ibn al-Ash'ath the first person to initiate experimental events in gastric physiology.[37]

According to Galen, in his work entitled *De ossibus ad tirones*, the lower jaw consists of two parts and it can be proven by the fact that it disintegrates in the middle when cooked.[7] Al-Baghdadi, while on a visit to Egypt, encountered many skeletal remains of those "who had died from starvation or had been eaten by their fellows" near Cairo.[7] He examined the skeletons and established that the mandible consists of one piece, not two as Galen had taught.[7] He wrote in his work *Al-Ifada w-al-Itibar fi al_Umar al Mushahadah w-al-Hawadith al-Muayanah bi Ard Misr*, or "Book of Instruction and Admonition on the Things Seen and Events Recorded in the Land of Egypt":[7]

> What I saw of this part of the corpses convinced me that the bone of the lower jaw is all one, with no joint nor suture. I have repeated the observation a great number of times, in over two thousand heads...I have been assisted by various different people, who have repeated the same examination, both in my absence and under my eyes...[7]

Unfortunately, Al-Baghdadi's discovery was ignored by any medical superiors or literature after his time. This was probably because the information was published in a book about the geography of Egypt.[7] The ignorance of this discovery could also have been because the medical establishment was not yet ready to give prominence to observation over the word of ancient authority.[7]

Drugs

Medical contributions made by Medieval Islam included the use of plants as a type of remedy or medicine. Medieval Islamic physicians used natural substances as a source of medicinal drugs—including *Papaver somniferum* Linnaeus, poppy, and *Cannabis sativa* Linnaeus, hemp.[38] In pre-Islamic Arabia, neither poppy nor hemp was known.[38] Hemp was introduced into the Islamic countries in the ninth century from India through Persia and Greek culture and medical literature.[38] The Greek, Dioscorides,[39] who according to the Arabs is the greatest botanist of antiquity, recommended hemp's seeds to "quench geniture" and its juice for earaches.[38] Beginning in 800 and lasting for over two centuries, poppy use was restricted to the therapeutic

realm.[38] However, the dosages often exceeded medical need and was used repeatedly despite what was originally recommended. Poppy was prescribed by Yuhanna b. Masawayh to relieve pain from attacks of gallbladder stones, for fevers, indigestion, eye, head and tooth aches, pleurisy, and to induce sleep.[38] Although poppy had medicinal benefits, Ali al-Tabari explained that the extract of poppy leaves was lethal, and that the extracts and opium should be considered poisons.[38]

Surgery

The development and growth of hospitals in ancient Islamic society expanded the medical practice to what is currently known as surgery. Surgical procedures were known to physicians during the medieval period because of earlier texts that included descriptions of the procedures.[1] Translation from pre-Islamic medical publishings was a fundamental building block for physicians and surgeons in order to expand the practice. Surgery was uncommonly practiced by physicians and other medical affiliates due to a very low success rate, even though earlier records provided favorable outcomes to certain operations.[1] There were many different types of procedures performed in ancient Islam, especially in the area of ophthalmology.

Techniques   Bloodletting and cauterization were techniques widely used in ancient Islamic society by physicians, as a therapy to treat patients. These two techniques were commonly practiced because of the wide variety of illnesses they treated. Cauterization, a procedure used to burn the skin or flesh of a wound, was performed to prevent infection and stop profuse bleeding. To perform this procedure, physicians heated a metal rod and used it to burn the flesh or skin of a wound. This would cause the blood from the wound to clot and eventually heal the wound.[40]

Bloodletting, the surgical removal of blood, was used to cure a patient of bad "humours" considered deleterious to one's health.[40] A phlebotomist performing bloodletting on a patient drained the blood straight from the veins. "Wet" cupping, a form of bloodletting, was performed by making a slight incision in the skin and drawing blood by applying a heated cupping glass. The heat and suction from the glass caused the blood to rise to the surface of the skin to be drained. "Dry cupping", the placement of a heated cupping glass (without an incision) on a particular area of a patient's body to relieve pain, itching, and other common ailments, was also used.[40] Though these procedures seem relatively easy for phlebotomists to perform, there were instances where they had to pay compensation for causing injury or death to a patient because of carelessness when making an incision. Both cupping and phlebotomy were considered helpful when a patient was sickly.[40]

Treatment Surgery was important in treating patients with eye complications, such as trachoma and cataracts. A common complication of trachoma patients is the vascularization of the tissue that invades the cornea of the eye, which was thought to be the cause of the disease, by ancient Islamic physicians. The technique used to correct this complication was done surgically and known today as peritomy. This procedure was done by "employing an instrument for keeping the eye open during surgery,a number of very small hooks for lifting, and a very thin scalpel for excision."[40] A similar technique in treating complications of trachoma, called pterygium, was used to remove the triangular-shaped part of the bulbar conjunctiva onto the cornea. This was done by lifting the growth with small hooks and then cut with a small lancet. Both of these surgical techniques were extremely painful for the patient and intricate for the physician or his assistants to perform.[40]

In medieval Islamic literature, cataracts were thought to have been caused by a membrane or opaque fluid that rested between the lens and the pupil. The method for treating cataracts in medieval Islam (known in English as couching) was known through translations of earlier publishings on the technique.[40] A small incision was made in the sclera with a lancet and a probe was then inserted and used to depress the lens, pushing it to one side of the eye. After the procedure was complete, the eye was then washed with salt water and then bandaged with cotton wool soaked in oil of roses and egg whites. After the operation, there was concern that the cataract, once it had been pushed to one side, would reascend, which is why patients were instructed to lie on his or her back for several days following the surgery.[40]

Anesthesia and antisepsis In both modern society and medieval Islamic society, anesthesia and antisepsis are important aspects of surgery. Before the development of anesthesia and antisepsis, surgery was limited to fractures, dislocations, traumatic injuries resulting in amputation, and urinary disorders or other common infections.[40] Ancient Islamic physicians attempted to prevent infection when performing procedures for a sick patient, for example by washing a patient before a procedure; similarly, following a procedure, the area was often cleaned with "wine, wined mixed with oil of roses, oil of roses alone, salt water, or vinegar water", which have antiseptic properties.[40] Various herbs and resins including frankincense, myrrh, cassia, and members of the laurel family were also used to prevent infections, although it is impossible to know exactly how effective these treatments were in the prevention of sepsis. The pain-killing uses of opium had been known since ancient times; other drugs including "henbane, hemlock, soporific

black nightshade, lettuce seeds" were also used by Islamic physicians to treat pain. Some of these drugs, especially opium, were known to cause drowsiness, and some modern scholars have argued that these drugs were used to cause a person to lose consciousness before an operation, as a modern day anesthetic would. However, there is no clear reference to such a use before the 16th century.[40]

Muslim scholars introduced mercuric chloride to disinfect wounds.[41]

3.7.6 Hospitals

Many hospitals were developed during the early Islamic era. They were called Bimaristan, which is a Persian word meaning "house [or place] of the sick."[42] The idea of a hospital being a place for the care of sick people was taken from the early Caliphs.[43] The bimaristan is seen as early as the time of Muhammad, and the Prophet's mosque in the city of Madinah held the first Muslim hospital service in its courtyard.[44] During the Ghazwah Khandaq (the Battle of the Trench), Muhammad came across wounded soldiers and he ordered a tent be assembled to provide medical care.[44] Over time, Caliphs and rulers expanded traveling bimaristans to include doctors and pharmacists.

Umayyad Caliph Al-Walid ibn Abd al-Malik is often credited with building the first bimaristan in Damascus in 707 AD.[45] The bimaristan had a staff of salaried physicians and a well equipped dispensary.[44] It treated the blind, lepers and other disabled people, and also separated those patients with leprosy from the rest of the ill.[44] Some consider this bimaristan no more than a *lepersoria* because it only segregated patients with leprosy.[45] The first true Islamic hospital was built during the reign of Caliph Harun al-Rashid.[43] The Caliph invited the son of chief physician, Jabril ibn Bukhtishu to head the new Baghdad bimaristan. It quickly achieved fame and led to the development of other hospitals in Baghdad.[43]

Features of bimaristans

As hospitals developed during the Islamic civilization, specific characteristics were attained. Bimaristans were secular. They served all people regardless of their race, religion, citizenship, or gender.[43] The Waqf documents stated nobody was ever to be turned away.[44] The ultimate goal of all physicians and hospital staff was to work together to help the well-being of their patients.[44] There was no time limit a patient could spend as an inpatient;[45] the Waqf documents stated the hospital was required to keep all patients until they were fully recovered.[43] Men and women were admitted to separate but equally equipped wards.[43][44] The separate wards were further divided into mental disease, contagious disease, non-contagious disease, surgery, medicine, and eye disease.[44][45] Patients were attended to by same sex nurses and staff.[45] Each hospital contained a lecture hall, kitchen, pharmacy, library, mosque and occasionally a chapel for Christian patients.[5][45] Recreational materials and musicians were often employed to comfort and cheer patients up.[45]

The hospital was not just a place to treat patients, it also served as a medical school to educate and train students.[44] Basic science preparation was learned through private tutors, self-study and lectures. Islamic hospitals were the first to keep written records of patients and their medical treatment.[44] Students were responsible in keeping these patient records, which were later edited by doctors and referenced in future treatments.[45]

During this era, physician licensure became mandatory in the Abbasid Caliphate.[45] In 931 AD, Caliph Al-Muqtadir learned of the death of one of his subjects as a result of a physician's error.[5] He immediately ordered his muhtasib Sinan ibn Thabit to examine and prevent doctors from practicing until they passed an examination.[5][45] From this time on, licensing exams were required and only qualified physicians were allowed to practice medicine.[5][45]

3.7.7 Pharmacy

The birth of pharmacy as an independent, well-defined profession was established in the early ninth century by Muslim scholars. Al-Biruni states that "pharmacy became independent from medicine as language and syntax are separate from composition, the knowledge of prosody from poetry, and logic from philosophy, for it [pharmacy] is an aid [to medicine] rather than a servant". Sabur (d. 869) wrote the first text on pharmacy.[46]

3.7.8 Women and medicine

During the medieval time period Hippocratic treaties became used widespread by medieval physicians, due the treaties practical form as well as their accessibility for medieval practicing physicians.[47] Hippocratic treaties of Gynecology and Obstetrics were commonly referred to by Muslim clinicians when discussing female diseases.[47] The Hippocratic authors associated women's general and reproductive health and organs and functions that were believed to have no counterparts in the male body.[47]

Beliefs

The Hippocratics blamed the womb for many of the women's health problems, such as schizophrenia.[47] They described the womb as an independent creature inside the female body; and, when the womb was not fixed in place by pregnancy, the womb which craves moisture, was believed to move to moist body organs such as the liver, heart, and brain.[47] The movement of the womb was assumed to cause many health conditions most particularly that of menstruation was also considered essential for maintaining women's general health.

Many beliefs regarding women's bodies and their health in the Islamic context can be found in the religious literature known as "medicine of the prophet." These texts suggested that men stay away from women during their menstrual periods, "for this blood is corrupt blood," and could actually harm those who come in contact with it.[48] Much advice was given with respect to the proper diet to encourage female health and in particular fertility. For example: quince makes a woman's heart tender and better; incense will result in the woman giving birth to a male; the consumption of water melons while pregnant will increase the chance the child is of good character and countenance; dates should be eaten both before childbirth to encourage the bearing of sons and afterwards to aid the woman's recovery; parsley and the fruit of the palm tree stimulates sexual intercourse; asparagus eases the pain of labor; and eating the udder of an animal increases lactation in women.[49] In addition to being viewed as a religiously significant activity, sexual activity was considered healthy in moderation for both men and women. However, the pain and medical risk associated with childbirth was so respected that women who died while giving birth could be viewed as martyrs.[50] The use of invocations to God, and prayers were also a part of religious belief surrounding women's health, the most notable being Muhammad's encounter with a slave-girl whose scabbed body he saw as evidence of her possession by the Evil Eye. He recommended that the girl and others possessed by the Eye use a specific invocation to God in order to rid themselves of its debilitating effects on their spiritual and physical health.[51]

Roles

It has been written that male guardians such as fathers and husbands did not consent to their wives or daughters being examined by male practitioners unless absolutely necessary in life or death circumstances.[52] The male guardians would just as soon treat their women themselves or have them be seen by female practitioners for the sake of privacy.[52] The women similarly felt the same way; such is the case with pregnancy and the accompanying processes such as child birth and breastfeeding, which were solely reliant upon advice given by other women.[52] The role of women as practitioners appears in a number of works despite the male dominance within the medical field. Two female physicians from

Ibn Zuhr's family served the Almohad ruler Abu Yusuf Ya'qub al-Mansur in the 12th century.[53] Later in the 15th century, female surgeons were illustrated for the first time in Şerafeddin Sabuncuoğlu's *Cerrahiyyetu'l-Haniyye* (*Imperial Surgery*).[54] The treatment provided of women by men was justified to some, whom were believers, through the ideals of the Prophetic medicine (al-tibba alnabawi) other wise known as "medicine of the prophet" (tibb al-nabi) which provided the argument that men can treat women, and women men, even if this means they must expose the patients genitals in necessary circumstances.[52]

Female doctors, Midwives, and wet nurses have all been mentioned in literature of the time period.[55]

3.7.9 Role of Christians

A hospital and medical training center existed at Gundeshapur. The city of Gundeshapur was founded in 271 by the Sassanid king Shapur I. It was one of the major cities in Khuzestan province of the Persian empire in what is today Iran. A large percentage of the population were Syriacs, most of whom were Christians. Under the rule of Khosrau I, refuge was granted to Greek Nestorian Christian philosophers including the scholars of the Persian School of Edessa (Urfa)(also called the Academy of Athens), a Christian theological and medical university. These scholars made their way to Gundeshapur in 529 following the closing of the academy by Emperor Justinian. They were engaged in medical sciences and initiated the first translation projects of medical texts.[56] The arrival of these medical practitioners from Edessa marks the beginning of the hospital and medical center at Gundeshapur.[57] It included a medical school and hospital (bimaristan), a pharmacology laboratory, a translation house, a library and an observatory.[58] Indian doctors also contributed to the school at Gundeshapur, most notably the medical researcher Mankah. Later after Islamic invasion, the writings of Mankah and of the Indian doctor Sustura were translated into Arabic at Baghdad.[59] Daud al-Antaki was one of the last generation of influential Arab Christian writers.

3.7.10 Legacy

Medieval Islam's receptiveness to new ideas and heritages helped it make major advances in medicine during this time, adding to earlier medical ideas and techniques, expanding the development of the health sciences and corresponding institutions, and advancing medical knowledge in areas such as surgery and understanding of the human body, although many Western scholars have not fully acknowledged its influence (independent of Roman and Greek in-

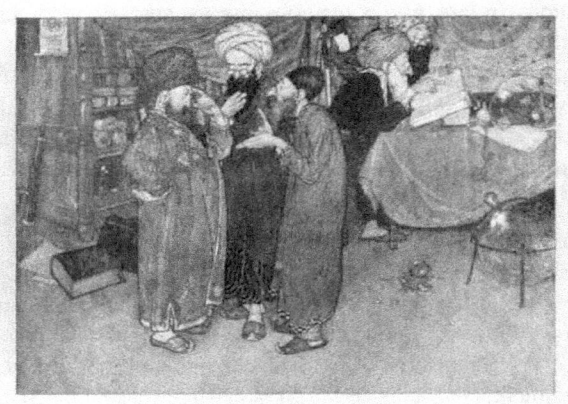

An illustration by Arthur Rackham from the 1001 Nights depicting medieval physicians.

fluence) on the development of medicine.[34]

Through the establishment and development of hospitals, ancient Islamic physicians were able to provide more intrinsic operations to cure patients, such as in the area of ophthalmology. This allowed for medical practices to be expanded and developed for future reference.

The contributions of the two major Muslim philosophers and physicians, Al-Razi and Ibn Sina, provided a lasting impact on Muslim medicine. Through their compilation of knowledge into medical books they each had a major influence on the education and filtration of medical knowledge in Islamic culture.

Additionally there were some iconic contributions made by women during this time, such as the documentation: of female doctors, physicians, surgeons, wet nurses, and midwives.

3.7.11 See also

- *Al-Tasrif*
- Anatomy Charts of the Arabs
- Bimaristan
- Ibn Sina Academy of Medieval Medicine and Sciences
- Inventions in the Islamic world
- Islamic Bioethics
- Islamic Golden Age
- Medieval medicine
- Science in the medieval Islamic world
- *De Gradibus*

- *Medical Encyclopedia of Islam and Iran*

- *The Canon of Medicine*

- Unani

- Prophetic medicine

3.7.12 Notes and references

Citations

[1] Pormann, Peter E.; Savage-Smith, Emilie (2007). *Medieval Islamic Medicine*. Edinburgh University Press. ISBN 0-7486-2066-4.

[2] Siraisi, Nancy G. (2001). *Medicine and the Italian universities 1250–1600*. Leiden: Brill. p. 203. ISBN 90-04-11942-6.

[3] Rassool, G.Hussein (2014). *Cultural Competence in Caring for Muslim Patients*. Palgrave Macmillan. pp. 90–91. ISBN 978-1-137-35841-7.

[4] D.o.H. p.50, As-Suyuti's Medicine of the Prophet p.125

[5] Shanks, Nigel J.; Dawshe, Al-Kalai (January 1984). "Arabian medicine in the Middle Ages" (PDF). *Journal of the Royal Society of Medicine* **77** (1): 60–65. PMC 1439563. PMID 6366229.

[6] Broumand, Behrooz. "The contribution of Iranian scientists to world civilization" (PDF). *Arch Iranian Med 2006* **9** (3): 288–290.

[7] Prioreschi, Plinio (2001). *A History of Medicine: Byzantine and Islamic medicine* (1st ed.). Omaha, NE: Horatius Press. p. 394. ISBN 1-888456-04-3.

[8] National Library of Medicine digital archives.

[9] Matthias Tomczak. "Lecture 11: Science, technology and medicine in the Roman Empire.". *Science, Civilization and Society (Lecture series)*.

[10] Saad, Bashar; Azaizeh, Hassan; Said, Omar (1 January 2005). "Tradition and Perspectives of Arab Herbal Medicine: A Review". *Evidence-Based Complementary and Alternative Medicine* **2** (4): 475–479. doi:10.1093/ecam/neh133. PMC 1297506. PMID 16322804.

[11] Saunders 1978, p. 193.

[12] Levey, Martin (1967). "Medical Ethics of Medieval Islam with Special Reference to Al-Ruhāwī's "Practical Ethics of the Physician"". *Transactions of the American Philosophical Society*. New Series (American Philosophical Society) **57** (3): 1–100. ISSN 0065-9746. JSTOR 1006137.

[13] Selin, Helaine, ed. (1997). *Encyclopaedia of the history of science, technology and medicine in non-western cultures*. Kluwer. p. 930. ISBN 0-7923-4066-3.

[14] Haque, Amber (2004). "Psychology from Islamic Perspective: Contributions of Early Muslim Scholars and Challenges to Contemporary Muslim Psychologists". *Journal of Religion and Health* **43** (4): 357–377 [361]. doi:10.1007/s10943-004-4302-z.

[15] Bazmee Ansari, A.S. (1976). "Abu Bakr Muhammad Ibn Yahya: Universal scholar and scientist". *Islamic Studies* **15** (3): 155–166. Retrieved 6 December 2011.

[16] W. Madelung (1 August 2011). "ALĪ AL-REŻĀ, the eighth Imam of the Emāmī Shiʿites.". *Iranicaonline.org*. Retrieved 18 June 2014.

[17] Staff writer. "The Golden time of scientific bloom during the Time of Imam Reza (A.S) (Part 2)". *Tebyan.net*. Retrieved 21 June 2014.

[18] Loudon, Irvine (2002-03-07). *Western Medicine: An Illustrated History*. Oxford University Press. p. 44. ISBN 9780199248131. Retrieved 12 September 2012.

[19] Karaman, Huseyin (June 2011). "Abu Bakr Al Razi (Rhazes) and Medical Ethics" (PDF). *Ondokuz Mayis University Review of the Faculty of Divinity* (30): 77–87. ISSN 1300-3003. Retrieved 1 December 2011.

[20] AL-RAZI article at Muslim Philosophy

[21] Deming, David (2010). *Science and Technology in World History: The ancient world and classical civilization*. Jefferson: Mcfarland. p. 93. ISBN 0-7864-3932-7.

[22] Tibi, Selma (April 2006). "Al-Razi and Islamic medicine in the 9th century". *Journal of the Royal Society of Medicine* **99** (4): 206–208. ISSN 0141-0768. Retrieved 6 December 2011.

[23] Rāzī, Abū Bakr Muḥammad ibn Zakarīyā. "The Comprehensive Book on Medicine - كتاب الحاوى فى الطب". *World Digital Library*. Retrieved 2014-03-02.

[24] "The Comprehensive Book on Medicine - كتاب الحاوي". *World Digital Library* (in Arabic). c. 1674. Retrieved 2014-03-02.

[25] Rāzī, Abū Bakr Muḥammad ibn Zakarīyā (1529). "The Comprehensive Book on Medicine - Continens Rasis". *World Digital Library* (in Latin). Retrieved 2014-03-02.

[26] Rāzī, Abū Bakr Muḥammad ibn Zakarīyā. "The Book of Medicine Dedicated to Mansur and Other Medical Tracts - Liber ad Almansorem". *World Digital Library* (in Latin). Retrieved 2014-03-02.

[27] Rāzī, Abū Bakr Muḥammad ibn Zakarīyā. "The Book on Medicine Dedicated to al-Mansur - الكتاب المنصوري في الطب". *World Digital Library* (in Amharic and Arabic). Retrieved 2014-03-02.

[28] "Commentary on the Chapter Nine of the Book of Medicine Dedicated to Mansur - Commentaria in nonum librum Rasis ad regem Almansorem". *World Digital Library* (in Latin). 1542. Retrieved 2014-03-02.

[29] Moosavi, Jamal (April–June 2009). "The Place of Avicenna in the History of Medicine". *Avicenna Journal of Medical Biotechnology* **1** (1). ISSN 2008-2835. Retrieved 7 December 2011.

[30] Colgan, Richard. *Advice to the Healer: On the Art of Caring.* Springer, 2013, p. 37.(ISBN 978-1-4614-5169-3)

[31] Sajadi, Mohammad M.; Davood Mansouri; Mohamad-Reza M. Sajadi (5 May 2009). "Ibn Sina and the Clinical Trial". *Annals of Internal Medicine* **150** (9): 640–643. doi:10.7326/0003-4819-150-9-200905050-00011. ISSN 0003-4819. Retrieved 7 December 2011.

[32] Huff, Toby (2003). *The Rise of Early Modern Science: Islam, China, and the West.* Cambridge University Press. p. 169. ISBN 0-521-52994-8.

[33] Savage-Smith, E. (1 January 1995). "Attitudes Toward Dissection in Medieval Islam". *Journal of the History of Medicine and Allied Sciences 50, no. 1* **50** (1): 67–110. doi:10.1093/jhmas/50.1.67. PMID 7876530.

[34] Hehmeyer, Ingrid; Khan Aliya (8 May 2007). "Islam's forgotten contributions to medical science". *Canadian Medical Association Journal* **176** (10): 1467. doi:10.1503/cmaj.061464. Retrieved 6 December 2011.

[35] A FORGOTTEN CHAPTER IN THE HISTORY OF THE CIRCULATION OF THE BLOOD Ann Surg. 1936 July; 104(1): 1–8

[36] Hannam, James (2011). *The Genesis of Science.* Regnery Publishing. p. 262. ISBN 1-59698-155-5.

[37] Haddad, Farid S. (18 March 2007). "Interventional physiology on the Stomach of aLive Lion: AlJ,mad ibn Abi ai-Ash'ath (959 AD)". *Journal of the Islamic Medical Association* **39**: 35. doi:10.5915/39-1-5269. Retrieved 4 December 2011.

[38] Hamarneh, Sami (July 1972). "Pharmacy in medieval islam and the history of drug addiction" (PDF). *Medical History* **16** (3): 226–237. doi:10.1017/s0025727300017725. PMC 1034978. PMID 4595520. Retrieved 4 December 2011.

[39] Forbes, Andrew ; Henley, Daniel; Henley, David (2013). 'Pedanius Dioscorides' in: *Health and Well Being: A Medieval Guide.* Chiang Mai: Cognoscenti Books. ASIN: B00DQ5BKFA 1953

[40] Pormann, Peter (2007). *Medieval Islamic medicine.* Washington, D.C.: Georgetown University Press. pp. 115–138.

[41] Maillard, Adam P. Fraise, Peter A. Lambert, Jean-Yves (2007). *Principles and Practice of Disinfection, Preservation and Sterilization.* Oxford: John Wiley & Sons. p. 4. ISBN 0470755067.

[42] Horden, Peregrine (Winter 2005). "The Earliest Hospitals in Byzantium, Western Europe, and Islam". *Journal of Interdisciplinary History* **35** (3): 361–389. doi:10.1162/0022195052564243.

[43] Nagamia, Hussain (October 2003). "Islamic Medicine History and Current Practice" (PDF). *Journal of the International Society for the History of Islamic Medicine* **2** (4): 19–30. Retrieved 1 December 2011.

[44] Rahman, Haji Hasbullah Haji Abdul (2004). "The development of the Health Sciences and Related Institutions During the First Six Centuries of Islam". *ISoIT*: 973–984.

[45] Miller, Andrew C (December 2006). "Jundi-Shapur, bimaristans, and the rise of academic medical centres". *Journal of the Royal Society of Medicine* **99** (12). pp. 615–617. doi:10.1258/jrsm.99.12.615.

[46] O'Malley, Charles Donald (1970). *The History of Medical Education: An International Symposium Held February 5-9, 1968, Volume 673.* Berkeley, Univ. of Calif. Press: University of California Press. pp. 60–61. ISBN 0520015789.

[47] Gadelrab, Sherry (2011). "Discourses on Sex difference in medieval scholarly Islamic thought". *Journal of History of Medicine and Allied Sciences* **66**.

[48] Cyril Elgood, "Tibb-Ul-Nabbi or Medicine of the Prophet," Osiris vol. 14, 1962. (selections): 60.

[49] Elgood, "Tibb-Ul-Nabbi or Medicine of the Prophet," 75, 90, 96, 105, 117.

[50] Elgood, "Tibb-Ul-Nabbi or Medicine of the Prophet," 172.

[51] Elgood, "Tibb-Ul-Nabbi or Medicine of the Prophet," 152-153

[52] Pormann, Peter (2009). "The Art of Medicine: female patients and practitioners in medieval Islam" (PDF). *Perspectives* **373**: 1598–1599. doi:10.1016/s0140-6736(09)60895-3. Retrieved 1 December 2011.

[53] "Islamic Culture and the Medical Arts: The Art as a Profession". United States National Library of Medicinedate=15 April 1998.

[54] Bademci, G (2006). "First illustrations of female "Neurosurgeons" in the fifteenth century by Serefeddin Sabuncuoglu" (PDF). *Neurocirugía* **17**: 162–165. doi:10.4321/s1130-14732006000200012.

[55] Shatzmiller, Mya (1994). *Labour in the Medieval Islamic World.* p. 353.

[56] *The American Journal of Islamic Social Sciences 22:2* Mehmet Mahfuz Söylemez, *The Jundishapur School: Its History, Structure, and Functions*, p.3.

[57] Gail Marlow Taylor, *The Physicians of Gundeshapur*, (University of California, Irvine), p.7.

[58] Cyril Elgood, *A Medical History of Persia and the Eastern Caliphate*, (Cambridge University Press, 1951), p.7.

[59] Cyril Elgood, *A Medical History of Persia and the Eastern Caliphate*, (Cambridge University Press, 1951), p.3.

Bibliography

- Morelon, Régis; Rashed, Roshdi (1996). *Encyclopedia of the History of Arabic Science* **3**. Routledge. ISBN 0-415-12410-7

- Browne (1862-1926), Edward G. (2002). *Islamic Medicine*. Goodword Books. ISBN 81-87570-19-9.

- Dols, Michael W. (1984). *Medieval Islamic Medicine: Ibn Ridwan's Treatise "On the Prevention of Bodily Ills in Egypt"*. Comparative Studies of Health Systems and Medical Care. University of California Press. ISBN 0-520-04836-9.

- Pormann, Peter E.; Savage-Smith, Emilie (2007). *Medieval Islamic Medicine*. Edinburgh University Press. ISBN 0-7486-2066-4.

- Porter, Roy (2001). *The Cambridge Illustrated History of Medicine*. Cambridge University Press. ISBN 0-521-00252-4.

- Saunders, John J. (1978). *A History of Medieval Islam*. Routledge. ISBN 978-0-415-05914-5.

- Ullmann, Manfred (1978). *Islamic Medicine*. Islamic Surveys **11**. Edinburgh: Univ. Press. ISBN 0-85224-325-1.

3.7.13   External links

- Islamic Medical Manuscripts at the National Library of Medicine.

- Arabic Medical Manuscripts at the UCL Centre for the History of Medicine.

- Islamic Culture and the Medical Arts at the National Library of Medicine.

- Influence On the Historical Development of Medicine by Prof. Hamed Abdel-reheem Ead.

- Al-Zahrawi (Albucasis) – A light in the Middle Ages in Europe by Dr. Sharif Kaf Al-Ghazal

- Contagion – Perspectives from Pre-Modern Societies

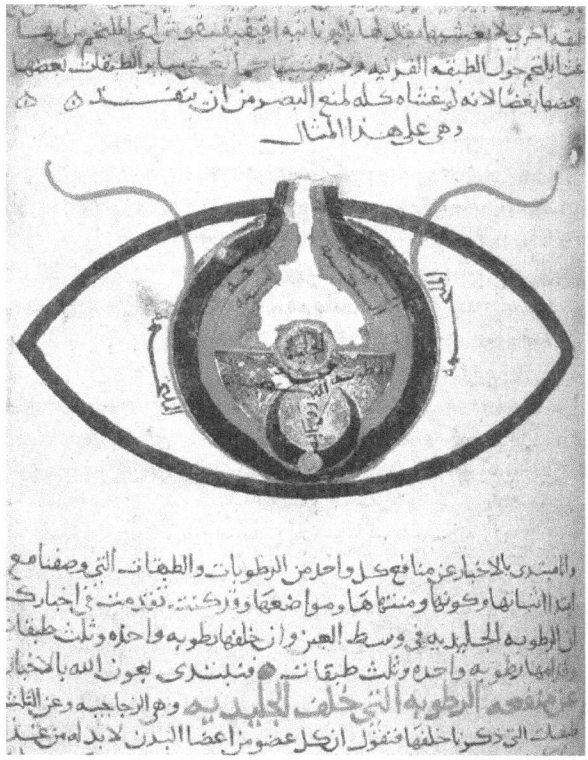

An Arabic manuscript, dated 1200CE, titled Anatomy of the Eye, *authored by al-Mutadibih.*

3.8   Ophthalmology in medieval Islam

Ophthalmology was one of the foremost branches **in medieval Islamic medicine**. The oculist or *kahhal* (كحال), a somewhat despised professional in Galen's time, was an honored member of the medical profession by the Abbasid period, occupying a unique place in royal households. Medieval Islamic scientists (unlike their classical predecessors) considered it normal to combine theory and practice, including the crafting of precise instruments, and therefore found it natural to combine the study of the eye with the practical application of that knowledge.[1] The specialized instruments used in their operations ran into scores. Innovations such as the "injection syringe", a hollow needle, invented by Ammar ibn Ali of Mosul, which was used for the extraction by suction of soft cataracts, were quite common.

Muslim physicians described such conditions as pannus, glaucoma (described as 'headache of the pupil'), phlyctenulae, and operations on the conjunctiva. They were the first to use the words 'retina' and 'cataract'.

3.8.1 Education and history

To become a practitioner, there was no one fixed method or path of training. There was even no formal specialization in the different branches of medicine, as might be expected. But some students did eventually approximate to a specialist by acquiring proficiency in the treatment of certain diseases or in the use of certain drugs.

Nevertheless, it was standard and necessary to learn and understand the works and legacy of predecessors. Among those one can mention, *The alteration of the eye* by Yuhanna ibn Masawayh, whose work can be considered the earliest work on Ophthalmology, followed by Hunain ibn Ishaq, known in the west as Johannitius, for his work *The ten treatises of the eye*.

Cataract extraction

The next major landmark text on ophthalmology was the *Choice of Eye Diseases* written in Egypt by the Iraqi Ammar bin Ali Al Mawsili who attempted the earliest extraction of cataracts using suction. He invented a hollow metallic syringe, which he applied through the sclerotic and successfully extracted the cataracts through suction. He wrote the following on his invention:

> "Then I constructed the hollow needle, but I did not operate with it on anybody at all, before I came to Tiberias. There came a man for an operation who told me: Do as you like with me, only I cannot lie on my back. Then I operated on him with the hollow needle and extracted the cataract; and he saw immediately and did not need to lie, but slept as he liked. Only I bandaged his eye for seven days. With this needle nobody preceded me. I have done many operations with it in Egypt."[2]

Other contributions

Avicenna, in *The Canon of Medicine* (c. 1025), described sight as one of the five external senses.[3] The Latin word "retina" is derived from Avicenna's Arabic term for the organ.[4]

In his *Coliget*, Averroes (1126–1198) was the first to attribute photoreceptor properties to the retina,[5] and he was also the first to suggest that the principle organ of sight might be the arachnoid membrane (*aranea*). His work led to much discussion in 16th century Europe over whether the principle organ of sight is the traditional Galenic crystalline humour or the Averroist *aranea*, which in turn led to the discovery that the retina is the principle organ of sight.[6]

Ibn al-Nafis wrote a large textbook on ophthalmology called *The Polished Book on Experimental Ophthalmology*. The book is divided into two sections: "On the Theory of Ophthalmology" and "Simple and Compunded Ophthalmic Drugs".[7] Other significant works in medieval Islamic ophthalmology include Rhazes' *Continens*, Ali ibn Isa al-Kahhal's *Notebook of the Oculists*, and the ethnic Assyrian Christian Jibrail Bukhtishu's *Medicine of the Eye*, among numerous others.

3.8.2 Ottoman Empire

In the Ottoman Empire, and well into the Republic of Turkey of the 20th century, a class of ambulatory eye surgeons, popularly known as the 'kırlangıç oğlanları' ('sons of the swallow') operated on cataract using special knives. From contemporary sources can be glimpsed that the reputation of these "blinding frauds" was far from spotless.[8]

3.8.3 Notes

[1] David C. Lindberg (1980), *Science in the Middle Ages*, University of Chicago Press, p. 21, ISBN 0-226-48233-2

[2] Finger, Stanley (1994), *Origins of Neuroscience: A History of Explorations Into Brain Function*, Oxford University Press, p. 70, ISBN 0-19-514694-8

[3] Finger, Stanley (1994), *Origins of Neuroscience: A History of Explorations Into Brain Function*, Oxford University Press, p. 71, ISBN 0-19-514694-8

[4] Finger, Stanley (1994), *Origins of Neuroscience: A History of Explorations Into Brain Function*, Oxford University Press, p. 69, ISBN 0-19-514694-8

[5] Martin-Araguz, A.; Bustamante-Martinez, C.; Fernandez-Armayor, Ajo V.; Moreno-Martinez, J. M. (2002). "Neuroscience in al-Andalus and its influence on medieval scholastic medicine", *Revista de neurología* **34** (9), p. 877-892.

[6] Lindberg, David C. (1981), *Theories of Vision from Al-kindi to Kepler*, University of Chicago Press, p. 238, ISBN 0-226-48235-9

[7] Albert Z. Iskandar, "Ibn al-Nafis", in Helaine Selin (1997), *Encyclopaedia of the History of Science, Technology, and Medicine in Non-Western Cultures*, Kluwer Academic Publishers, ISBN 0-7923-4066-3.

[8] Laban Kaptein (ed.), Ahmed Bican, *Dürr-i meknûn*, p. 31f. Asch 2007. ISBN 978-90-902140-8-5

3.8.4 References

- Ibn Abi Usaybi'ah, Uyun ul-Inba' fi Tabaqat ul-Atibba, Cairo 1882.

- Nizami Arudhi, Chahar Maqalah. Gibb Series. London, 1921.

- Zeylessouf-ed-douleh, Matrah ul-anzār. Tabriz, 1916.

- Bar Hebraeus, *Historia Dynastiarum*, Edward Pococke's edition, Oxford 1663.

- M. Brett, W. Foreman. The Moors: Islam in the west. 1980.

- Cyril Elgood. A Medical history of Persia and the eastern caliphate : the development of Persian and Arabic medical sciences, from the earliest times until the year A.D. 1932. 1979.

- Casey Wood. Memorandum book of a tenth-century oculist for the use of modern ophthalmologists : a translation of the Tadhkirat of Ali ibn Isa of Baghdad (cir. 940-1010 CE).

3.8.5 See also

- Islamic medicine

- Islamic science

- Islamic Golden Age

- List of Arab scientists and scholars

- List of Iranian scientists and scholars

3.9 Plague doctor costume

The **plague doctor's costume** was the clothing worn by a plague doctor to protect him from airborne diseases. The costume, originating in the 17th century, consisted of an ankle length overcoat and a bird-like beak mask often filled with sweet or strong smelling substances (commonly lavender), along with gloves, boots, a brim hat, and an outer over-clothing garment.[2]

3.9.1 Description

The mask had glass openings for the eyes and a curved beak shaped like that of a bird. Straps held the beak in front of the doctor's nose.[3] The mask had two small nose holes and was a type of respirator which contained aromatic items. [4] The beak could hold dried flowers (including roses and carnations), herbs (including mint), spices, camphor, or a vinegar sponge.[5][6] The purpose of the mask was to keep away bad smells, which were thought to be the principal cause of the disease in the miasma theory of infection, before it was

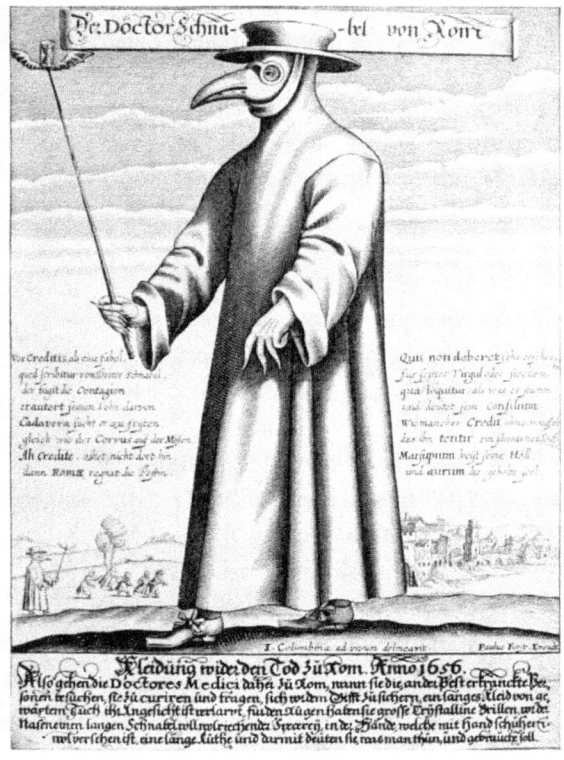

Paul Fürst, engraving, c. 1721, of a plague doctor of Marseilles (introduced as 'Dr Beaky of Rome'). His nose-case is filled with herbal material to keep off the plague.[1]

disproved by germ theory.[2][3] Doctors believed the herbs would counter the "evil" smells of the plague and prevent them from becoming infected.[3]

The beak doctor costume worn by plague doctors had a wide-brimmed leather hat to indicate their profession.[2][7] They used wooden canes to point out areas needing attention and to examine patients without touching them.[8] The canes were also used to keep people away,[9] to remove clothing from plague victims without having to touch them, and to take a patient's pulse.[2][10]

3.9.2 History

Medical historians have attributed the invention of the "beak doctor" costume to Charles de Lorme, who adopted in 1619 the idea of a full head-to-toe protective garment,[11] modeled after a soldier's armour.[12] This consisted of a bird-like mask and a long leather (Moroccan or Levantine)[12] or waxed-canvas gown which was from the neck to the ankle.[11][13][14] The over-clothing garment, as well as leggings, gloves, boots, and a hat, were made of waxed leather.[15] The garment was impregnated with similar fragrant items as the beak mask.[16] The costume may have older roots as some authors have described fourteenth-century plague doctors as wearing bird-like masks.[17][18][19]

This popular seventeenth century poem describes the plague doctor's costume.[20][21]

> As may be seen on picture here,
> In Rome the doctors do appear,
> When to their patients they are called,
> In places by the plague appalled,
> Their hats and cloaks, of fashion new,
> Are made of oilcloth, dark of hue,
> Their caps with glasses are designed,
> Their bills with antidotes all lined,
> That foulsome air may do no harm,
> Nor cause the doctor man alarm,
> The staff in hand must serve to show
> Their noble trade where'er they go.[22]

The Genevese physician Jean-Jacques Manget, in his 1721 work *Treatise on the Plague* written just after the Great Plague of Marseille, describes the costume worn by plague doctors at Nijmegen in 1636-1637. The costume forms the frontispiece of Manget's 1721 work.[23] The plague doctors of Nijmegen also wore beaked masks. Their robes, leggings, hats, and gloves were made of morocco leather.[24]

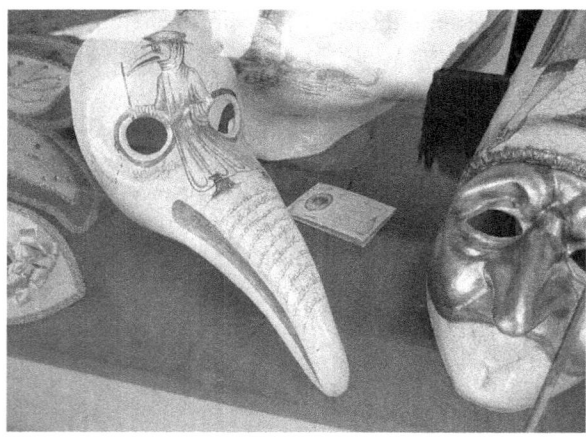

A beaked Venetian carnival mask with the inscription Medico della Peste *('Plague doctor') beneath the right eye*

This costume was also worn by plague doctors during the Plague of 1656, which killed 145,000 people in Rome and 300,000 in Naples.[25] The costume terrified people because it was a sign of imminent death. Plague doctors wore these protective costumes in accordance with their agreements when they attended their plague patients.

3.9.3 Culture

The costume is also associated with a *commedia dell'arte* character called *Il Medico della Peste* (the Plague Doctor), who wears a distinctive plague doctor's mask.[26] The Venetian mask was normally white, consisting of a hollow beak and round eye-holes covered with clear glass, and is one of the distinctive masks worn during the Carnival of Venice.[27]

3.9.4 References

Footnotes

[1] Füssli's image is reproduced and discussed in Robert Fletcher, *A tragedy of the Great Plague of Milan in 1630* (Baltimore: The Lord Baltimore Press, 1898), p. 16–17.

[2]
- Pommerville (Body Systems), p. 15
- Bauer, p. 145
- Abrams, p. 257
- Byfield, p. 26
- Glaser, pp. 33-34

[3] Ellis, p. 202

[4]
- Time-Life Books, pp. 140, 158
- Dolan, p. 139
- Ellis, p. 202
- Paton
- Martin, p. 121
- Sherman, p. 162
- Turner, p. 180
- Mentzel, p. 86
- Glaser, p. 36
- Hall, p. 67
- Infectious Diseases Society of America, Volume 11, p. 819
- Grolier, p. 700

[5] O'Donnell, p. 135

[6] Stuart, p. 15

[7] Center for Advanced Study in Theatre Arts, p. 83

[8] Doktor Schnabel von Rom, engraving by Paul Fürst (after J Columbina), Rome 1656.

[9] American Medical Association - *JAMA.: The Journal of the American Medical Association,* Volume 34, p. 639

[10] Pommerville, p. 9

[11] Boeckl, p. 15

[12] Carmichael, p. 57

[13] Carmichael, A.G. (2009), "Plague, Historical", in Schaechter, Moselio, *Encyclopedia of Microbiology* (3rd ed.), Elsevier, pp. 58–72, doi:10.1016/B978-012373944-5.00311-4

[14] Iqbal Akhtar Khan (May 2004). "Plague: the dreadful visitation occupying the human mind for centuries". *Transactions of the Royal Society of Tropical Medicine and Hygiene* **98** (5): 270–277. doi:10.1016/S0035-9203(03)00059-2. Charles Delorme (1584—1678), personal physician to King Louis XIII, was credited with introducing special protective clothing for plague doctors during the epidemic in Marseilles. It consisted of a beak-like mask supplied with aromatic substance, presumed to act as filter against the odour emanating from the patients, and a loose gown covering the normal clothing. On occasions, a drifting fragrance such as camphor was used.

[15] • Pommerville (Body Systems), p. 15
     • Hirts, p. 66
     • Reynolds, p. 23

[16] Kenda, p. 154

[17] *Geographical: the monthly magazine of the Royal Geographical Society*, Volume 63, April 1991, p. 19, *Plague doctors of the 14th century wore distinctive bird-like masks and were known as beak doctors.*

[18] • Pommerville (Body Systems), p. 15
     • Ellis, p.202
     • Byrne (Encyclopedia), p. 505
     • Sandler, p. 42
     • Paton
     • Ulrich's Periodicals Directory, ulrichsweb.com or email *magazine at geographical.co.uk,* Content Type : Academic / Scholarly

[19] Time-Life Books, p. 158 *Beak Doctor: during the Black Plague, a medical man who wore a bird mask to protect himself against infection.* Black plague definition: *In 14th-century Europe, the victims of the "black plague" had bleeding below the skin (subcutaneous hemorrhage) which made darkened ("blackened") their bodies. Black plague can lead to "black death" characterized by gangrene of the fingers, toes, and nose. Black plague is caused by a bacterium (Yersinia pestis) which is transmitted to humans from infected rats by the oriental rat flea..* medterm.com

[20] THE PLAGUE DOCTOR

[21] G. L. Townsend, "The Plague Doctor", *J Hist Med Allied Sci*, 20 (1965), 276. (The image is on p. 277).

[22] • Nohl, pp. 94, 95
     • Sandler, p. 42
     • Goodnow, p. 132

     • Walker, p. 96

[23] Manget, p. 3

[24] Timbs, p. 360

[25] The Plague Doctor

[26] Killinger, p. 95

[27] Carnevale

Works cited

• Abrams, J. J., *The Road Not Taken*, Simon and Schuster, 2005, ISBN 1-4169-2483-3

• Bauer, S. Wise, *The Story of the World Activity Book Two: The Middle Ages : From the Fall of Rome to the Rise of the Renaissance*, Peace Hill Press, 2003, ISBN 0-9714129-4-4

• Boeckl, Christine M., *Images of plague and pestilence: iconography and iconology*, Truman State Univ Press, 2000, ISBN 0-943549-85-X

• Byfield, Ted, *Renaissance: God in Man, A.D. 1300 to 1500: But Amid Its Splendors, Night Falls on Medieval Christianity*, Christian History Project, 2010, ISBN 0-9689873-8-9

• Byrne, Joseph Patrick, *Encyclopedia of Pestilence, Pandemics, and Plagues*, ABC-CLIO, 2008, ISBN 0-313-34102-8

• Carmichael, Ann G., "SARS and Plagues Past", in *SARS in Context: Memory, history, policy*, ed. by Jacalyn Duffin and Arthur Sweetman McGill-Queen's University Press, 2006, ISBN 0-7735-3194-7

• Center for Advanced Study in Theatre Arts, *Western European stages*, Volume 14, CASTA, 2002,

• Dolan, Josephine, *Goodnow's History of Nursing* , W. B. Saunders 1963 (Philadelphia and London), Library of Congress No. 16-25236

• Ellis, Oliver Coligny de Champfleur, *A History of Fire and Flame*, London: Simkin, Marshall, 1932; repr. Kessinger, 2004, ISBN 1-4179-7583-0

• Goodnow, Minnie, *Goodnow's history of nursing* , W.B. Saunders Co., 1968, OCLC Number: 7085173

• Glaser, Gabrielle, *The Nose: A Profile of Sex, Beauty, and Survival* , Simon and Schuster, 2003, ISBN 0-671-03864-8

- Grolier Incorporated, *The Encyclopedia Americana,* Volume 8; Volume 24, Grolier Incorporated, 1998, ISBN 0-7172-0130-9

- Hall, Manly Palmer, *Horizon,* Philosophical Research Society, Inc., 1949

- Hirst, Leonard Fabian, *The conquest of plague: a study of the evolution of epidemiology,* Clarendon Press, 1953,

- Infectious Diseases Society of America, *Reviews of infectious diseases,* Volume 11, University of Chicago Press, 1989

- Kenda, Barbara, *Aeolian winds and the spirit in Renaissance architecture: Academia Eolia revisited,* Taylor & Francis, 2006, ISBN 0-415-39804-5

- Killinger, Charles L., *Culture and customs of Italy,* Greenwood Publishing Group, 2005, ISBN 0-313-32489-1

- Nohl, Johannes, *The Black Death: A Chronicle of the Plague,* J. & J. Harper Edition 1969, Library of Congress No. 79-81867

- Manget, Jean-Jacques, *Traité de la peste recueilli des meilleurs auteurs anciens et modernes,* Geneva, 1721, online as PDF, 28Mb download

- Martin, Sean, *The Black Death,* Book Sales, 2009, ISBN 0-7858-2289-5

- Mentzel, Peter, *A traveller's history of Venice ,* Interlink Books, 2006, ISBN 1-56656-611-8

- O'Donnell, Terence, *History of life insurance in its formative years,* American Conservation Company, 1936

- Paton, Alex, "Cover image", *QJM: An International Journal of Medicine,* 100.4, 4 April 2007. (A commentary on the issue's cover photograph of The Posy Tree, Mapperton, Dorset.)

- Pommerville, Jeffrey, *Alcamo's Fundamentals of Microbiology: Body Systems,* Jones & Bartlett Learning, 2009, ISBN 0-7637-6259-8

- Pommerville, Jeffrey, *Alcamo's Fundamentals of Microbiology,* Jones & Bartlett Learning, 2010, ISBN 0-7637-6258-X

- Reynolds, Richard C., *On doctor[i]ng: stories, poems, essays, Simon and Schuster, 2001, ISBN 0-7432-0153-1*

- Sandler, Merton, *Wine: a scientific exploration,* CRC Press, 2003, ISBN 0-415-24734-9

- Sherman, Irwin W., *The power of plagues,* Wiley-Blackwell, 2006, ISBN 1-55581-356-9

- Stuart, David C., *Dangerous garden: the quest for plants to change our lives,* frances lincoln ltd, 2004, ISBN 0-7112-2265-7

- Timbs, John, *The Mirror of literature, amusement, and instruction,* Volume 37, J. Limbird, 1841

- Time-Life Books, *What life was like in the age of chivalry: medieval Europe, AD 800-1500,* 1997

- Turner, Jack, *Spice: The History of a Temptation ,* Random House, 2005, ISBN 0-375-70705-0

- Walker, Kenneth, *The story of medicine ,* Oxford University Press, 1955

3.10 Prophetic medicine

Prophetic medicine ('Al-Tibb al-nabawī, Arabic: الطب النبوي) refers to the actions and words (*hadith*) specifically of the Islamic prophet Muhammad with regards to sickness, treatment and hygiene, and the genre of writings undertaken primarily by non-physician scholars to collect and explicate these traditions.[1] It is distinct from Islamic medicine, in that the latter is a broader category encompassing a variety of medical practices rooted in Greek natural philosophy. Prophetic medical traditions exhort humans to not simply stop at following Muhammad's teachings, but encourage them to search for cures as well. The literature of Prophetic medicine thus occupies a symbolic role in the elucidation of Islamic identity as constituted by a particular set of relationships to science, medicine, technology and nature. There has historically been a tension in the understanding of the medical narratives: are they of the same nature as Muhammad's religious pronouncements, or are they time-sensitive, culturally-situated, and thus not representative of a set of eternal medical truths? [2] This body of knowledge was fully articulated only in the 14th century, at which point it was concerned with reconciling *Sunnah* (traditions) with the foundations of the Galenic humoral theory that was prevalent at the time in the medical institutions of the Islamicate world.[3] It is nonetheless a tradition with continued modern-day currency, as suggested by the online presence of resources on the genre.[4]

3.10.1 Overview

Prophetic medicine is sometimes casually identified with *Unani* medicine or traditional medicine, although it is distinguished from some iterations of these and from scientific medicine most predominantly by the former being specifi-cally a collection of advice attributed to Muhammad in the Islamic tradition.[5] One would do well to note that medieval interpretations of the medical hadith were produced in a Galenic medical context, while modern-day editions might bring in recent research findings to frame the importance of the genre. In the hadith, Muhammad recommended the use of honey and *hijama* (wet cupping) for healing and had generally opposed the use of cauterization for causing "pain and menace to a patient".[6] Other items with beneficial effects attributed to Muhammad, and standard features on traditional medicine in the Islamicate world, include olive oil; dates; *miswak* as a necessity for oral health and Nigella sativa or "black seed" or "black cumin" and its oils. These items are still sold in Islamic centers or sellers of other Islamic goods. The value of honey is traced to specific mention of its virtues in the Quran and not just Muhammad:

> And thy Lord taught the Bee to build its cells
> in hills, on trees, and in (men's) habitations;
> Then to eat of all the produce (of the earth), and
> find with skill the spacious paths of its Lord:
> there issues from within their bodies a drink
> of varying colours, wherein is healing for men:
> verily in this is a Sign for those who give thought.
> — Quran, sura 16 (An-Nahl), ayat 68-69[7]

Muhammad's firm belief in the existence of a cause and a cure for every disease is described in many hadith along the lines of the below:[6][8]

> Make use of medical treatment, for Allah
> has not made a disease without appointing a
> remedy for it, with the exception of one disease,
> namely old age.
> — Abu Dawood, *Sunan Abu Dawood*[9]

This belief can be said to be a grounding philosophy of this otherwise loosely-defined field,[10] and is said to have encouraged early Muslims to engage in medical research and seek out cures for diseases known to them.[8]

3.10.2   Works

While the prominent works focused on treatment of the hadith related to health date from several centuries A.H., *Sahih al-Bukhari* and other earlier collections included these as well. 'Abd Allah b. Bustâm al-Nîsâbûrî's Tlbb al-a'imma, aggregating a legacy of several Shi'ite Imams, is widely considered to be the first known treatise on Prophetic medicine, although it is rooted in a somewhat different

cosmology.[2] The canonical al-Bukhari corpus, divided into 97 books with 3450 chapters,includes over a 100 traditions in its book 76 loosely related to medicine, covering topics ranging from precautions against leprosy and epidemics to the forbidding of alcohol and suicide. The most notable works that still survive[11] are attributed to religious scholars and largely not to Galenic physicians, although the latter are occasionally referenced.

Ibn Qayyim Al-Jawziyya in the 1300s produced one of the most influential works about prophetic medicine in his 277-chapter book, *Al-Tibb al-Nabawiyy*. Al-Jawziyya deals with a diversity of treatments as recommended by Muhammad but also engages with ethical concerns, discussing malpractice and the hallmarks of the competent doctor.[12] Ethics of medical practice continue to be an important marker of Islamic medicine for some.[13] Al-Jawziyya also elaborates on the relationship between medicine and religion.[1]

A theologian renowned for his exegetical endeavors, Al-Suyuti also composed two works on prophetic medicine, one of which was on sexual relations as ordered by Muhammad.[12] Al-Suyuti's other manuscript divides medicine into 3 types: traditional, spiritual and preventive (e.g. dietary regimen and exercise). Along with Al-Jawziyya, Al-Suyuti also included commentary that spoke to dealing with contagion and thus was relevant to the Black Death in the Islamic world.

Both of the works above also address bioethical issues of abortion and conception, issues that, like the idea of Islamic medical heritage as being holistic, continue to be important in constructions of modern Islamic identity.[14] Other notable works include those of Ibn Tulun (d. AD 1546) and Al-Dhahabi (d. AD 1348).

3.10.3   References

[1] Muzaffar Iqbal, Science and Islam (Westport, CT: Greenwood press,2007),59

[2] Ahmed Ragab. Journal of the American Oriental Society 132.4 (2012). 657-673.

[3] Stearns, Justin (1 December 2011). "Writing the History of the Natural Sciences in the Pre-modern Muslim World: Historiography, Religion, and the Importance of the Early Modern Period". *History Compass* **9** (12): 923–951. doi:10.1111/j.1478-0542.2011.00810.x.

[4] Tibb-e-Nabawi ~ Healing by ISLAM, both for the body & soul, for the doctor & patient, for the sick & healthy; Prophetic-Medicine

[5] Rosenthal, Franz; Marmorstein, Jenny (1975). *The classical heritage in Islam*. Berkeley: University of California Press. p. 182. ISBN 0-520-01997-0.

[6] Deuraseh Nurdeen. "Ahadith of the Prophet on Healing in Three Things (al-Shifa' fi Thalatha): An Interpretational". *Journal of the International Society for the History of Islamic Medicine* **2003** (4): 14–20.

[7] Quran 16:69

[8] Borchardt, John K. (2002). "Arabic Pharmacy during the Age of the Caliphs". *Drug News & Perspectives* **15** (6): 383. doi:10.1358/dnp.2002.15.6.840036.

[9] Sunan Abu Dawood, 28:3846

[10] Irmeli Pehro, The Prophet's Medicine: A Creation of the Muslim Traditionalist Scholars (Helsinki: Kokemaki, 1995)

[11] The Magic of Science

[12] Cyril Elgood (1962) The Medicine Of the Prophet. PubMed Central, 146-153.

[13] Islamic medicine on the rise in Southeast Asia

[14] Fazlur Rahman Health and Medicine in the Islamic Tradition: Change and Identity. (New York : Crossroad, 1987)

3.10.4 Further reading

- Ghaly, Mohammed, *Prophetic Medicine,* in Muhammad in History, Thought, and Culture: An Encyclopedia of the Prophet of God (2 vols.), Edited by C. Fitzpatrick and A. Walker, Santa Barbara, ABC-CLIO, 2014, Vol. II, pp.502-506. ISBN 1610691776

3.10.5 External links

- U.S. National Library of Medicine: Prophetic Medicine

- International Institute of Islamic Medicine

3.11 Psychology in medieval Islam

Islamic psychology or **'Ilm al-Nafs**[1] (Arabic, علم النفس), the science of the *Nafs* ("self" or "psyche"),[2] refers to the medical and philosophical study of the psyche from an Islamic perspective and addresses topics in psychology, neuroscience, philosophy of mind, and psychiatry as well as psychosomatic medicine.

Concepts from medieval Islamic thought have been reexamined by Muslim psychologists and scholars in the 20th and 21st centuries.[3]

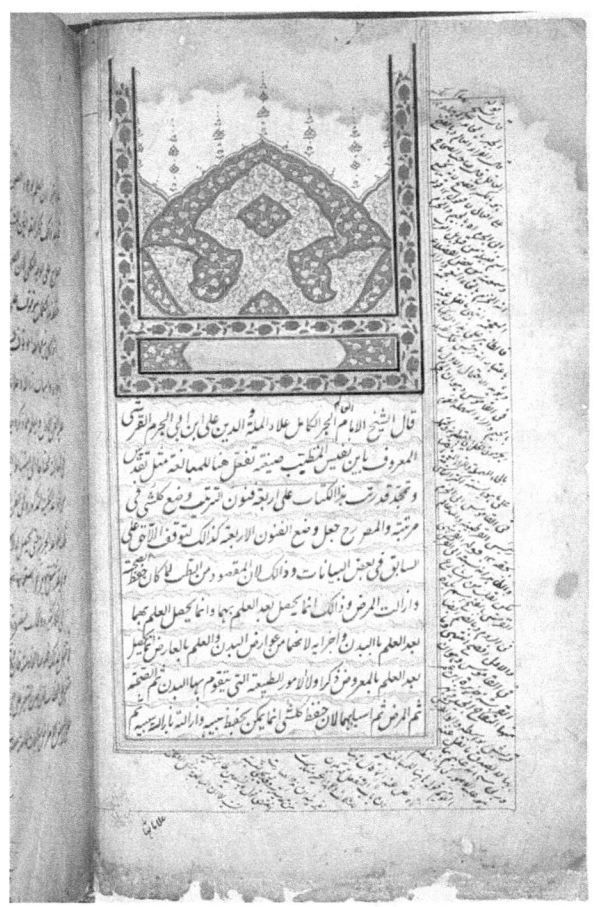

A medical work by Ibn al-Nafis, who corrected some of the erroneous theories of Galen and Avicenna on the anatomy of the brain.

3.11.1 Terminology

In the writings of Muslim scholars, the term *Nafs* (self or soul) was used to denote individual personality and the term *fitrah* for human nature. *Nafs* encompassed a broad range of faculties including the *qalb* (heart), the *ruh* (spirit), the *aql* (intellect) and *irada* (will). Muslim scholarship was strongly influenced by Greek and Indian philosophy as well as by the study of scripture, drawing particularly from Galen' understanding of the four humors of the body.

In medieval Islamic medicine in particular, the study of mental illness was a speciality of its own,[4] and was variously known as *al-'ilaj al-nafs* (approximately "curing/treatment of the ideas/soul/vegetative mind),[5] *al-tibb al-ruhani* ("the healing of the spirit," or "spiritual health") and *tibb al-qalb* ("healing of the heart/self," or "mental medicine").[2]

The Classical Arabic term for the mentally ill was "majnoon" which is derived from the term "Janna", which means "covered". It was originally thought that mentally ill individuals could not defferentiate between the real and the unreal, however, due to their nuanced nature treatment on the mentally ill could not be generalized as it was in medieval Europe [6] This term was gradually redefined among the educated, and was defined by Avicenna as "one who suffers from a condition in which reality is replaced with fantasy".

3.11.2 Ethics and Theology

In the Islamic world, special legal protections were given to the mentally ill. This attitude was reinforced by scripture, as exemplified in Sura 4:5 of the Qur'an:

"Do not give your property which God assigned you to manage to the insane: but feed and clothe the insane with this property and tell splendid words to them."[4]

This Quranic verse summarized Islam's attitudes towards the mentally ill, who were considered unfit to manage property but must be treated humanely and be kept under care by either a guardian or the state.[4]

3.11.3 Major Contributors

Muhammad ibn Zakariya al-Razi

Muhammad ibn Zakariya al-Razi (865 – 925), known as Rhazes in the western tradition, was an influential Persian physician, philosopher, and scientist during the Golden Age of Islam, and among the first in the world to write on mental illness and psychotherapy.[7] As chief physician of Baghdad hospital, he was also the director of one of the first psychiatric wards in the world. Two of his works in particular, *El-Mansuri* and *Al-Hawi*, provide descriptions and treatments for mental illnesses.[7]

Abu-Ali al-Husayn ibn Abdalah ibn-Sina

Abu-Ali al-Husayn ibn Abdalah ibn-Sina (980-1030), known to the west as Avicenna, was a Persian polymath who is widely regarded for his writings on such diverse subjects as philosophy, physics, medicine, mathematics, geology, Islamic theology, and poetry. In his most widely celebrated work, the Canon of Medicine (Al-Qanun-fi-il-Tabb), he provided descriptions and treatments for such conditions as insomnia, mania, vertigo, paralysis, stroke, epilepsy, and depression as well as male sexual dysfunction. He was a pioneer in the field of psychosomatic medicine, linking changes in mental state to changes in the body.[8]

3.11.4 Mental Healthcare

The Golden Age of Islam was unique in that treatment of mental disorders was carried out in hospitals. Psychiatric hospitals were constructed in Baghdad in 705 and Cairo in 805, and there is evidence to suggest that there was also one such facility in operation Fez during the 8th century.[7]

Treatment of Mental Illness

In addition to medication, treatment for mental illness might include baths, music, and occupational therapy reflecting the great emphasis placed on the relationship between illness of the mind and problems in the body. Medicine would be prescribed in order to re-balance the four humors of the body, an imbalance of which might result in psychosis.[8] Insomnia, for example, was thought to result from excessive amounts of the dry humors which could be remedied by the use of humectants.

3.11.5 See also

- Islamic philosophy

- Medicine in the medieval Islamic world

- Ophthalmology in medieval Islam

- Science in medieval Islam

3.11.6 Notes

[1] (Haque 2004, p. 358)

[2] Deuraseh, Nurdeen; Mansor Abu, Talib (2005), "Mental health in Islamic medical tradition", *The International Medical Journal* **4** (2): 76–79.

[3] (Haque 2004)

[4] (Youssef, Youssef & Dening 1996, p. 58)

[5] (Haque 2004, p. 376)

[6] Okasha, A. (2001), "Egyptian Contribution to the Conception of Mental Health", *Eastern Mediterranean Health Journal* **7** (3): 377–380.

[7] Wael Mohamed, C.R. (2012). "Arab and Muslim Contributions to Modern Neuroscience". *International Brain Research Organization History of Neuroscience*.

[8] A. Okasha, C.R. (1). "Mental Health and Psychiatry in the Middle East". *Eastern Mediterranean Health Journal* **7**: 336–347. Check date values in: |date= (help)

3.11.7 References

- Haque, Amber (2004), "Psychology from Islamic Perspective: Contributions of Early Muslim Scholars and Challenges to Contemporary Muslim Psychologists", *Journal of Religion and Health* **43** (4): 357–377, doi:10.1007/s10943-004-4302-z

- Plott, C. (2000), *Global History of Philosophy: The Period of Scholasticism*, Motilal Banarsidass, ISBN 81-208-0551-8

- Youssef, Hanafy A.; Youssef, Fatma A.; Dening, T. R. (1996), "Evidence for the existence of schizophrenia in medieval Islamic society", *History of Psychiatry* **7** (25): 55–62, doi:10.1177/0957154X9600702503, PMID 11609215

Chapter 4

Text and image sources, contributors, and licenses

4.1 Text

- **Medieval medicine of Western Europe** *Source:* https://en.wikipedia.org/wiki/Medieval_medicine_of_Western_Europe?oldid=691122414 *Contributors:* Edward, Paul Barlow, Sannse, Ahoerstemeier, Adam Bishop, Reddi, Zoicon5, Jeeves, Optim, Ebricca, Wetman, Hajor, Robbot, RedWolf, Mr-Natural-Health, Inter, Nunh-huh, Tom harrison, Marcika, Monedula, Everyking, Rpyle731, Erich gasboy, Fergananim, Antandrus, Xandar, John Foley, Pmanderson, Beginning, Kevin Rector, D6, Perey, Discospinster, Rich Farmbrough, Dbachmann, Stbalbach, Bender235, ESkog, Brian0918, CanisRufus, Bletch, Shanes, Bobo192, Stesmo, Smalljim, Polylerus, DanielVallstrom, Auriel~enwiki, Snowolf, Ringbang, Dreadnought1906, Mindmatrix, TigerShark, SDC, Mandarax, Graham87, Magister Mathematicae, Rjwilmsi, Quiddity, Camdic, Nihiltres, Sanbeg, Nivix, RexNL, KFP, Akhenaten0, King of Hearts, DVdm, Bgwhite, Phantomsteve, RussBot, Gaius Cornelius, Veledan, Rjensen, Dureo, Renata3, Dspradau, Allens, Bluezy, Luk, MaeseLeon, SmackBot, Jagged 85, Canthusus, Srnec, Apers0n, Peter Isotalo, Gilliam, Hmains, Chris the speller, Bluebot, Persian Poet Gal, Hurdygurdyman1234, Dlohcierekim's sock, Baa, Colonies Chris, Can't sleep, clown will eat me, Leinad-Z, Aquarius Rising, Quartermaster, Rrburke, Iblardi, Kukini, Cyberevil, John, AmiDaniel, Makyen, BranStark, NativeForeigner, Delta x, Ytny, Tawkerbot2, Ale jrb, Eric, Gregbard, MVNdude, SyntaxError55, Michaelas10, Tawkerbot4, Chrislk02, Lo2u, Thijs!bot, Epbr123, Daniel, John254, Bobblehead, Dawnseeker2000, AntiVandalBot, Seaphoto, Mary Mark Ockerbloom, Res2216firestar, Justinhwang1996, DuncanHill, Magioladitis, Pharillon, VoABot II, R.E.S.A., Wikidudeman, Doug Coldwell, Phunting, DerHexer, Supahfreekeh, MartinBot, Wtrploplyr1000, MNAdam, Nono64, Trusilver, Bandersnatch42, Bogey97, Demonic dark angel, Johnbod, NewEnglandYankee, Cometstyles, Grendlefuzz, WardXmodem, Jeter888888, Dchall1, Clarince63, LeaveSleaves, BigDunc, Insanity Incarnate, Sfmammamia, SieBot, Scarian, WereSpielChequers, Karaboom, Keilana, Wilson44691, Bsherr, Techman224, KathrynLybarger, ClueBot, The Thing That Should Not Be, ImperfectlyInformed, Senzangakhona, SuperHamster, Arjayay, Qqwwwwwwww, Razorflame, Catalographer, Aitias, Versus22, Cowsflyhi, Rpm93, Spitfire, Gnowor, Casewicz, MystBot, Queenmomcat, Fluffernutter, Ka Faraq Gatri, MrOllie, Quietmarc, Hintss, Luckyseven10, Tide rolls, Lightbot, OlEnglish, Dmitry Rozhkov, Yobot, ArchonMagnus, Jim1138, Pyrrhus16, Piano non troppo, Bezio, Clarinetguy097, Kingpin13, Ulric1313, ImperatorExercitus, Citation bot, Wsmith2008, G-Baby94, Env laser, Frosted14, Sjcj1969, N419BH, A.amitkumar, FrescoBot, Jprulestheworld01, Lhawkings, Kobrabones, Intelligentsium, DrilBot, I dream of horses, Vrenator, Miracle Pen, Weedwhacker128, TimONeill, DARTH SIDIOUS 2, ChanDMan2010, Crazydumdum, Gfs6grade, Nbcd, Fwgibbs, Salvio giuliano, EmausBot, John of Reading, Orphan Wiki, Acather96, WikitanvirBot, Razor2988, Moswento, St. Brigit, Hashemi1971, Azuris, Thefirstwizard, DASHBotAV, Rocketrod1960, ClueBot NG, Inkowik, MelbourneStar, Escapepea, Widr, Lizzie9000, Sauer119, KLBot2, BG19bot, PhnomPencil, Snow Blizzard, BattyBot, Torvalu4, Khazar2, Dexbot, Lugia2453, Watchme1, Loverofthelight, Samuelbekoe5, Hoppeduppeanut, Monkbot, Ephemeratta, Saladjames, Scor97, Kalah.arellanes, Cameron2200, Federico Leva (BEIC), Ign christian, Blueray6, Rhbuckner and Anonymous: 349

- **Black Death** *Source:* https://en.wikipedia.org/wiki/Black_Death?oldid=690747330 *Contributors:* AxelBoldt, Magnus Manske, TwoOneTwo, Kpjas, Derek Ross, LC~enwiki, David Parker, Joakim Ziegler, Mav, Zundark, The Anome, Koyaanis Qatsi, Taw, Pinkunicorn, Malcolm Farmer, Jagged, Danny, Rmhermen, SimonP, Graft, Montrealais, Ewen, Olivier, Someone else, Rickyrab, Stevertigo, Spiff~enwiki, D, Kwertii, Llywrch, Voidvector, Dominus, Jahsonic, Kku, Liftarn, Gabbe, Ixfd64, Zeno Gantner, Sannse, AlexR, Yann, Minesweeper, Looixx~enwiki, Mkweise, Ahoerstemeier, Pjamescowie, William M. Connolley, Muriel Gottrop~enwiki, G-Man, CatherineMunro, Darkwind, Gem~enwiki, Harry Wood, Julesd, Glenn, Error, Rossami, Scott, Andres, Evercat, Smack, Mechanolatry, Uriber, RodC, Adam Bishop, Janko, Mw66, Piolinfax, IceKarma, DJ Clayworth, CBDunkerson, Tpbradbury, Maximus Rex, Taxman, LMB, VeryVerily, SEWilco, Shizhao, Topbanana, Wetman, Jusjih, Cvaneg, David.Monniaux, Pollinator, Jeffq, Earl Manchester, Ben Hateva, Branddobbe, Rolando, Chris 73, Simonf, Sanders muc, Swestrup, Donreed, Yelyos, Romanm, Naddy, Lowellian, Sverdrup, Academic Challenger, Puckly, Flauto Dolce, Rursus, Ojigiri~enwiki, Auric, Gidonb, Humus sapiens, Diderot, Caknuck, Catbar, Hadal, Dehumanizer, Saforrest, Wikibot, Nerval, Benc, Demerzel~enwiki, Cautious, Neckro, Xanzzibar, Wayland, Cordell, Rik G., Giftlite, JamesMLane, Unother, DocWatson42, MPF, Marnanel, Fennec, Jyril, Akadruid, Haeleth, Whitti, Nunh-huh, Fennario, Tom harrison, Lupin, Ferkelparade, Malcontent, Obli, Bradeos Graphon, Peruvianllama, Everyking, No Guru, Curps, Michael Devore, Henry Flower, MingMecca, Varlaam, Revth, Guanaco, Eequor, SWAdair, Mckaysalisbury, Bobblewik, Deus Ex, Golbez, OldakQuill, Fergananim, Utcursch, SoWhy, Andycjp, Nova77, Geni, Antandrus, Williamb, OverlordQ, Bcameron54, Cjewell, Ro4444, ShakataGaNai, Jossi, Dunks58, Rdsmith4, Oneiros, The Land, OwenBlacker, DragonflySixtyseven, Sebbe, Bumm13, Kevin B12, Bencoland, M.e, Icairns, Jmf1205, Bk0, Sam Hocevar, TiMike, Neutrality, Imjustmatthew, Ukexpat, Dcandeto, Kevyn, M1ss1ontomars2k4, Adashiel,

Trevor MacInnis, Rculatta, Lacrimosus, Glasperlenspiel, Kate, Gazpacho, Zro, Mike Rosoft, Ouro, Freakofnurture, DanielCD, Jim Henry, Jkl, Discospinster, ElTyrant, 4pq1injbok, Rich Farmbrough, KillerChihuahua, Rhobite, C12H22O11, Qutezuce, Vsmith, Mecanismo, BalowStar, Bishonen, Eric Shalov, Xezbeth, Dbachmann, Justwes, Pavel Vozenilek, Paul August, Stereotek, SpookyMulder, Stbalbach, Bender235, Rubicon, ESkog, Sc147, Kbh3rd, Kaisershatner, Lalala666, Dpotter, RJHall, CanisRufus, Mr. Billion, El C, Aude, Shanes, Spearhead, Linkoman, Sietse Snel, RoyBoy, Triona, Nrbelex, Wareh, Jpgordon, Rlaager, Bobo192, Longhair, Feitclub, Smalljim, Reinyday, Cmdrjameson, Reuben, Mytildebang, Cayte, Thanos6, Rockhopper10r, La goutte de pluie, Xrx2007, Jojit fb, Nk, Bdamokos, The Recycling Troll, MPerel, Sam Korn, (aeropagitica), Polylerus, Ultra megatron, Klhuillier, Merope, Storm Rider, Patsw, Mrzaius, Alansohn, Gary, Anthony Appleyard, Uncle.bungle, Tek022, Megan 189, Atlant, Rd232, Jeltz, Wouterstomp, Riana, Wikidea, AzaToth, MarkGallagher, Goldom, Lightdarkness, Viridian, InShaneee, WikiParker, Malo, Svartalf, Snowolf, CaseInPoint, TaintedMustard, KingTT, Shogun~enwiki, Yuckfoo, Docboat, Evil Monkey, RainbowOfLight, Sciurinæ, Shoefly, Mikeo, Dominic, Pfahlstrom, Bsadowski1, Alai, Ghirlandajo, Pymander, HGB, Tainter, Bookandcoffee, KTC, Ceyockey, Dismas, Kevin Hayes, Gmaxwell, Paradiver, Boothy443, Richard Arthur Norton (1958-), Kelly Martin, The JPS, OwenX, TigerShark, Camw, LOL, Muya, Unixer, AdashRASH, Commander Keane, JBellis, Jeff3000, MONGO, SynOP, Kelisi, Kmg90, Schzmo, Trevor Andersen, Jleon, Scootey, GregorB, Snagari, SDC, Plrk, SeventyThree, Wayward, 쾅쾅쾅쾅쾅, Alan Canon, Karam.Anthony.K, Bebenko, Dysepsion, MrSomeone, GSlicer, Tslocum, Ashmoo, Graham87, WBardwin, Magister Mathematicae, Kbdank71, Bunchofgrapes, FreplySpang, RxS, Jclemens, Grammarbot, Mendaliv, Kane5187, Corambis, Canderson7, Solace098, BruceW07, Sjakkalle, Rjwilmsi, Angusmclellan, Crazyvas, Panoptical, Vary, Papayoung, Marasama, Hiberniantears, Tangotango, Tawker, SMC, Stilgar135, Crazynas, Kalogeropoulos, Graibeard, Jkeaton, Bhadani, DoubleBlue, Sango123, Oo64eva, Yamamoto Ichiro, Algebra, Bash, RainR, Titoxd, Wegsjac, SchuminWeb, Kammerbulle, Musical Linguist, Nihiltres, Crazycomputers, Harmil, Who, Itinerant1, Isotope23, JYOuyang, NekoDaemon, Andy85719, Gparker, RexNL, Nickhap, Gurch, Wars, Egthegreat, TheDJ, President Rhapsody, Algri, Fresheneesz, Salvadorjo~enwiki, Kevinhksouth, Silivrenion, Sairen42, Chobot, DJProFusion, Chwyatt, Ahpook, Cactus.man, Digitalme, Gwernol, The Rambling Man, Kombucha, Retaggio, RattusMaximus, Sceptre, Jimp, Wolfmankurd, Midgley, Phantomsteve, RussBot, Jtkiefer, Anonymous editor, Conscious, Kevs, Zafiroblue05, Ilai, Splash, Pigman, GLaDOS, DanMS, Groogle, SpuriousQ, Nesbit, Hydrargyrum, Stephenb, Lord Voldemort, Gaius Cornelius, Ironist, CambridgeBayWeather, Ihope127, Dsmouse, Wimt, GeeJo, MarcK, Shanel, NawlinWiki, NicolasDelerue, Dysmorodrepanis~enwiki, Wiki alf, BGManofID, LaszloWalrus, Jaxl, Rjensen, Bongoed, Space man333, Dureo, Thiseye, Bmdavll, Irishguy, Nick, Saoshyant, Brandon, Banes, Brian Crawford, Cholmes75, Tommaisey, Rmky87, Envoypv, Desk Jockey, Raven4x4x, Waqas1987, Davidpk212, Misza13, Semperf, Tony1, Hinto, DGJM, Aaron Schulz, Todfox, Killercat, Drumsac, DeadEyeArrow, Paaskynen, Rayc, Robot Monk, Wolfling, Ajarmst, Alpha 4615, Fabiob~enwiki, Efbrazil, Max Schwarz, Wknight94, Bob247, Jcvamp, Jkelly, Pawyilee, FF2010, AnnaKucsma, MLA, Emijrp, Theodolite, TarenCapel, Ali K, Silverhorse, Chase me ladies, I'm the Cavalry, Theda, Closedmouth, Ketsuekigata, Peoplez1k, Fang Aili, Pb30, Abune, Youssef51, BorgQueen, JoanneB, Symon, Fram, Peter, JLaTondre, RenamedUser jaskldjslak904, Xil, ArielGold, Katieh5584, Kungfuadam, Junglecat, Banus, Thomas Blomberg, Rikimaru~enwiki, NeilN, Phil071391, Airconswitch, Nippoo, DVD R W, Luk, Joshbuddy, A bit iffy, Cafe Nervosa, SmackBot, Kellen, Reedy, Prodego, KnowledgeOfSelf, Olorin28, Hydrogen Iodide, Itsme12690, Gfunkdave, Pgk, Longlostmariobro, Felix Dance, Blue520, WilyD, Sfsdfd, Jagged 85, Davewild, Mscuthbert, Anastrophe, Jedikaiti, Oben, Delldot, Hardyplants, Kmwalke, StefanoC, PJM, CGameProgrammer, Brossow, Geoff B, Srnec, TantalumTelluride, Commander Keane bot, Yamaguchi쾅쾅, Marxtone, PeterSymonds, Peter Isotalo, Gilliam, Brianski, Portillo, Donama, Hmains, Ghosts&empties, Skizzik, Dspserpico, Icemuon, Durova, Schmiteye, Saros136, Izehar, Chris the speller, Happywaffle, Timbouctou, Timmy son, Taelus, Persian Poet Gal, Lepetitvagabond, Ian13, MK8, Thumperward, Snori, IanBailey, Kemet, Fluri, SchfiftyThree, Droll, Moshe Constantine Hassan Al-Silverburg, RayAYang, Kevin Ryde, Leoni2, The Moose, Colonies Chris, Oatmeal batman, Rlevse, Gracenotes, D-Rock, Can't sleep, clown will eat me, Shalom Yechiel, Leinad-Z, Jinxed, Musculus~enwiki, AltGrendel, Furby100, OrphanBot, Onorem, Surfcuba, Avb, W377!M, Jbhood, TheKMan, Xiner, Pevarnj, GeorgeMoney, HBow3, Addshore, Flubbit, Whpq, RedHillian, Jmlk17, Piroroadkill, Flyguy649, Tsop, BostonMA, CZMJ, Runningidiot, AdamWeeden, Nakon, TedE, John D. Croft, EVula, Dreadstar, Lpgeffen, Falconeer, G-J, SeanAhern, Jon Awbrey, J y p, Latebird, Zzorse, Sturm, Richard0612, Deiz, Ck lostsword, Pilotguy, FelisLeo, Kukini, Carlosp420, Qmwne235, LanternLight, Drunken Pirate, Ceoil, Ohconfucius, EMan32x, Nishkid64, Eliyak, Rory096, Robomaeyhem, Swatjester, C 1, Ozhiker, Johncatsoulis, Harryboyles, Kuru, John, Fremte, Ian Spackman, Tazmaniacs, Jaganath, Sir Nicholas de Mimsy-Porpington, Stattouk, JorisvS, HonestTom, Zarniwoot, Vesperholly, A. Parrot, BillFlis, Slakr, Special-T, Stwalkerster, Lampman, Davemcarlson, Planninefromouterspace, Mr Stephen, Gum foil, Fedallah, Xiaphias, MegaMan2OO6, Waggers, Don Alessandro, Jstupple7, Sijo Ripa, Serlin, Barrek5, Winvirus, Citicat, Symposiarch, H, Thelastemperor, Myself0101, Mohamed Abdel Mageed, Vagary, Darry2385, Hectorian, Amitch, Roulette36, DabMachine, Norm mit, Keith-264, SimonD, Compboy1, Iridescent, Paulsuckow, Kencf0618, Profsnow, MobileOak, MIckStephenson, JoeBot, IvanLanin, Vocaro, Twas Now, Provocateur, MJO, CapitalR, Blehfu, Quodfui, Supertigerman, Gaybo%, Az1568, Courcelles, Chovain, Scarlet Lioness, Tawkerbot2, Tommysimpson, Timrem, Chris55, Flubeca, Capt Jack Doicy, ChrisCork, Joemcnulty, Orangutan, Herr chagall, CalebNoble, Idols of Mud, Yuheng, JForget, Redcoat-Mic, RWhite, Liam Skoda, CmdrObot, Tamoroso, Porterjoh, NKSCF, Ale jrb, Aaronak, Smably, Bhree, 0zymandias, Nunquam Dormio, CWY2190, Ruslik0, Stbodie, GHe, Jsmaye, Dgw, Goatchurch, Avillia, The Indigo Lemon, Casper2k3, Neelix, Gogogaga, Richard Keatinge, Tim1988, Tex, Nnp, Lau42, Nauticashades, Rudjek, Creek23, Doctormatt, Cydebot, Norwegianzealot, Wiki sosa, Kirkesque, Nergal-Behemoth, Grahamec, Steel, Gogo Dodo, Red Director, Jon Stockton, Bazzargh, Nohope, Master son, Katherine Tredwell, He Who Is, Dynaflow, DumbBOT, Chrislk02, Otm~enwiki, Inhumer, Optimist on the run, Garik, Kozuch, Stevenmahal, Ike-bana, Omicronpersei8, JodyB, Daniel Olsen, General Veers, Luka Krstulović, Rocket000, Saintrain, Benny1boy93, Alexthebam, FrancoGG, SummonerMarc, Malleus Fatuorum, Thijs!bot, Epbr123, Daa89563, Jpark3909, Kro666, LeeG, Jmg38, Sagaciousuk, Josephseagullstalin, Voracious reader, Andyjsmith, Mtdew24541, Ksimmons8888, PierceG, Oliver202, Luigifan, Pjvpjv, John254, A3RO, SomeStranger, Itsmejudith, Bernadettehuron, Artydude, Strausszek, Eilev G. Myhren~enwiki, Zuzana~enwiki, Notmyrealname, CPBOOTH, Khorshid, CharlotteWebb, Alaraxis, Thedarkestshadow, Northumbrian, Mentifisto, Hmrox, KrakatoaKatie, Cyclonenim, AntiVandalBot, Majorly, Luna Santin, QuiteUnusual, Bsimmons87, Carolmooredc, Fyunck(click), Doc Tropics, Jj137, TimVickers, Shadow girl, Clamster5, Darklilac, Gdo01, Spencer, Oddity-, Gpardo13, Blair Bonnett, Perakhantu, AtikuX, Muani, Ani td, Gökhan, Obeattie, Golgofrinchian, JAnDbot, Xhienne, Husond, MER-C, Andrewericoleman, Nthep, Agrestis, Speculoos, Instinct, Jonemerson, Db099221, Midnightdreary, Andonic, Igodard, Hut 8.5, Frankie816, Time3000, Dream Focus, Wimstead, Kerotan, GrimRepr39, Acroterion, Repku, Bencherlite, Lester Long, Moni3, Freedomlinux, Pedro, Bongwarrior, VoABot II, Mondebleu, Hb2019, MartinDK, Ishikawa Minoru, Dekimasu, Fusionmix, CC Guns, Davidjk, Kuyabribri, JamesBWatson, Shark slayer1028, Ling.Nut, Doug Coldwell, Glaurung quena, Lucyin, Rami R, Dinosaur puppy, WilliamFrancais, Aksmth, Thernlund, Animum, Kiwimandy, 28421u2232nfenfcenc, Boffob, Harrison keith, Allstarecho, MapMaster, Jagan no Otoko, Guayl, Dustiescott, Cpl Syx, Chris G, DerHexer, JaGa, Indianstar, Jodi.a.schneider, Zonemind, Textorus, Patstuart, Antissimo, DancingPenguin, Quidnunc, Theprowier, Jasonater, Pacemaster, Hdt83, MartinBot, Willjay, Mitch1209, Tobor0, Cheifsguy, Die Romantic, Rettetast, Juansidious, More-Ron, Jay Litman, Glossando, Burnedthru, R'n'B, CommonsDelinker, AlexiusHoratius, Fconaway, PrestonH, Dudley Miles, Jacobst, Discboy, Dinkytown, AlphaEta, J.delanoy, N00bFragger, DrKay, Trusilver, Bigcheesepie, Spathaky, Robert Bridson Cribb, Boghog, Uncle Dick, Cymbalta, Maurice Carbonaro, MrBell, Eliz81, NerdyNSK, Jasper33, OttoMäkelä, Icseaturtles, Maproom, Skullketon, Mrfunnyd, Johnbod, MagicMan78, McSly, Ignatzmice, Tidus9605605, Grosscha, Chelbabe, Aboutmovies, TheTrojanHought, Mikael Häggström, Blubba112, Skier Dude, Hillock65, Chumpdog85, Gurchzilla, Sonofu, WebHamster, Dmitri Yuriev, AntiSpamBot, (jarbarf), Spinach Dip, Illiterate11, Shomroni, Alexb102072, Moosetophat, Belovedfreak, NewEnglandYankee, Molly-in-md, Matthardingu, Hennessey, Patrick, SJP, Touch Of Light, Malerin, Olegwiki, Cometstyles, Alyssa hoffel, Tiggerjay, Remember the dot, Jamesofur, Talia May, Gwen Gale, LordCo Centre, Vanished user 39948282, Mike V, Kvdveer, Bawlix, Gtg204y, SuperWikipediaMaster, Randygonz, Emu bob 09, Duck71, HereItIs-Now, ZenobieG, Puyomaster, Useight, SD Hog rider, CA387, Omc, RjCan, Martial75, Gabriel bahena, Xiahou, Chris Item, CardinalDan, Richard New Forest, MattIzzy, Idioma-bot, Spellcast, Speciate, Fishmonkey45, Sumo su, Hugo999, PACKRATDC3, Zomgblah, Gothbag, Deor, CWii, Thedjatclubrock, Murderbike, Jeff G., Dqeswn, Alexandria, AlnoktaBOT, Ph8l, VasilievVV, Sirmelle~enwiki, Engelhardt, Meth-Man47, Barneca, Philip Trueman, Jsgw, Zeuron, TXiKiBoT, Cyclone77, Cosmic Latte, MeStevo, Hydra351, Bluetrombonist, PsychicKid1, Vipinhari, Myles325a, Pojanji, Philforhumanity, IMSancho, Eherot, Jank123456, Fifa2007~enwiki, Nrswanson, Anonymous Dissident, Ivan Viehoff, ElinorD, Gwinva, Sean D Martin, NVO, Qxz, Someguy1221, Billybobbobobbo, Rawrimalizard, Killjoy966, Anna Lincoln, Lradrama, Andrein, Brada Vang, Drpetersonthesecond, Martin451, Sirkad, Sanfranman59, Mzmadmike, Shiltermann, LeaveSleaves, Rhysdrummer, Philfaebuckie, Mannafredo, Cremepuff222, Nicholas.goder, Saturn star, Madhero88, Junnepy, Andrewaskew, Kilmer-san, IL7Soulhunter, Cantiorix, Synthebot, Falcon8765, Billy4, Wikidan829, KUHoopsfan247, Burntsauce, Seresin, Spinningspark, CoralWhite, Brianga, Truthanado, Dg-bzkg, Monty845, Chickyfuzz14, HiDrNick, Dessymona, Bubblylizzie, CT Cooper, Deconstructhis, LOTRrules, Glst2, Newbyguesses, Kolsen5, Awils1, Lord 1284, SieBot, Madman, Brenont, Sonicology, 4wajzkd02, Tiddly Tom, Graham Beards, Moonriddengirl, Scarian, M31n1k0v, Krawi, Katman4, Callipides~enwiki, Isil lome elda, Caltas, Westville man, Iloveyouxxxscar, Cwkmail, Ashkani, RJaguar3, MeegsC, Vanished User 8a9b4725f8376, Epeen2007, Cheezy8, JerrySteal, Merotoker1, Fibo1123581321, Nummer29, Arda Xi, Keilana, Mais2, Interchange88, Iames, Aillema, Flyer22 Reborn, Tiptoety, Radon210, Exert, Killer989, Andr987, Belinrahs, Oda Mari, Wilson44691, Snideology, GrayAngel007, Hzh, Bsherr, Ayudante, Dominik92, Oxymoron83, Byrialbot, Faradayplank, Avnjay, Nuttycoconut, Baseball Bugs, Lightmouse, Mjkhfg, Abdowiki, DMNT, Poindexter Propellerhead, Archaeogenetics, Ealdgyth, Jooy20, Yamaka122, Alex.muller, Psychosomatic Tumor, Peulle, Svick, Dravecky, Spitfire19, Belligero, N96, Spartan-James, Cyfal, Mad Hlaine Larkin, Witchkraut, Yair rand, Geoff Plourde, Dabomb87, Hordaland, Midx1004, DRTllbrg, Escape Orbit, A.C. Norman, Hadseys, 07sanjk, Lrmauro, 1sanj1, Mr. Granger, Faithlessthewonderboy, Atif.t2, MenoBot, Martarius, Apuldram, ClueBot, Dreist, Kl4m, Binksternet, Hot Shot Cheetor, Fyyer, Marcus Khoudair, Dobermanji, The Thing That Should Not Be, Patricklikewoah, Rjd0060, Michcomte, AnneBoleyn1536, EoGuy, Dean Wormer, Mafuyu~enwiki, Parkjunwung, Gegabone, Triguera, Acer1056, Arakunem, Saddhiyama, Hornet35, RJ88888, Anubis 009, Der Golem, Sungame, Koolbart, Skäpperöd, A lepa, CounterVandalismBot, Gigsta and tiger, VanessaCop, Niceguyedc, Derekristow, Richerman, Harland1, LizardJr8, TheSmuel, Steewi, Pyro0757, Neverquick, Cirt, Jeremiestrother, Margewel, Manishearth, Tanketz, DragonBot, Clayton hiller, AppleXpieXisXgod, Excirial, SeanQuinlan, Jaimelinternet, Anonymous101, Jusdafax, Crywalt, Tall Terry, Jefflayman, Mangafreak32, CrazyChemGuy, Diplodoc, Tornadou, Tiniti, Wikitumnus, The sock farmer, Abcdaaa1, Arcot, Bauer 1046, Gtstricky, Sivico, MorrisRob, Muhandes, Twinkle301, Vivio Testarossa, Lartoven, Austin2009, Mgdurand, Deqon, Ninja5624, NuclearWarfare, Redbullgivesuwind, Promethean, Jonjames1986, Gtman908, Gemstar140, NakanoHito, CowboySpartan, Scog, Jonnyboy706, Kaiba, Joeproszek, Razorflame, Deletionists are ruining Wiki-pedia, Jarjar9, Revotfel, Dangerboi, SchreiberBike, Audaciter, Polly, ChrisHodgesUK, Thehelpfulone, La Pianista, Catalographer, Thingg, Darren23, Aitias, 7, Subash.chandran007, Zombie433, Sarahisgay, Hwalee76, Robotjj, Jonker~enwiki, Micman, Cookiehead, SoxBot III, Egmontaz, Editor2020, Party, TEN10X, RJPe, BoBlanckenburg, SteelMariner, Life of Riley, Remembermetomorrow, XLinkBot, ChrisG4019, Joke1229, Nathan Johnson, Gonzonoir, Misterman4312, Utkarshshah007, Rror, Feinoha, Laurips, Avoided, Facts707, Cadege, WikHead, Appius Psychopompos~enwiki, Wahrhaft, Clam-man2000, Mluppino878, Saintmesmin, Paul1967, Rkarl13, Alexius08, Spoonkymonkey, Mm40, Sonyray, Psychward1234, Atomicdor, Asidemes, ZooFari, Tunda9605, Cublue, Kaleidoscope xtina, Good Olfactory, Airplaneman, Pat42143, Ejosse1, Thatguyflint, Surtsicna, Deineka, Bazj, Addbot, 11341134a, Galinkin, Shadowclad, DOI bot, Dawynn, Jojhutton, Acdriske, OmgItsTheSmartGuy, Trasman, Ronhjones, Fieldday-sunday, TheMatty, Vishnava, CanadianLinuxUser, Proxima Centauri, Chamal N, Reaperman, The Shadow-Fighter, Glane23, Henkt, Φοίνιξ, Chzz, Debresser, Roux, The hobo next door, Favonian, Doniago, LemmeyBOT, LinkFA-Bot, 5 albert square, Elen of the Roads, Тиверополник, Peridon, Skarlath, Hereford, Blurpflargblech, Vikaszt, Tide rolls, Lightbot, Jim the Dragon, Krano, Phreed100, QuadrivialMind, Gail, Ghostchick123, Dannywucu482, Alfie66, Frehley, DyingToRace, Ben Ben, Luckas-bot, KenshinHolstein, Dillardjj, Yobot, 2D, JohnnyCalifornia, Tohd8BohaithuGh1, Kushiban, Rsquire3, Victoriaearle, Leastminor, PMLawrence, Matanya, ᏂᎤᏂ, Rbwik, Matty, AnomieBOT, Letuño, SaaHc2B, Hairhorn, Netanand, Rockypedia, Floozybackloves, Piano non troppo, Terrykwon, Tom87020, Kingpin13, Flewis, Bluerasberry, Materialscientist, Living001, RobertEves92, Mcvittal, ImperatorExercitus, Ckruschke, Citation bot, Srinivas, OllieFury, Goteamben, E2eamon, Maiella, Neurolysis, Ssbb5, LilHelpa, Goresh, Xqbot, Altoff, Sketchmoose, Historicist, Toctocwilly, Poopmypoop, Gonzagol, Jsima016, Biweee11, Ederek, The Banner, Ronaldoisaplayer, Oppolord, Rootef, Wikiaisj, Arghiamsupermanman, Gigemag76, Stalkerperson, Poetaris, Pontificalibus, Jeffrey Mall, Mononomic, Rajkotia, Br77rino, Onrswan, Frosted14, MilfordBoy991, Shirik, Kurtdriver, Foreverprovence, RibotBOT, Edwardsesq, Carrite, Shiver of recognition, Amaury, Tombuk1, Sabrebd, GhalyBot, Shadowjams, Sesu Prime, Pauswa, Green Cardamom, RetiredWikipedian789, FrescoBot, Ash1299, Fortdj33, Tobby72, Saintgeorge2, Grand-Duc, Sky Attacker, JuniperisCommunis, Cargoking, Dger, Finalius, Jamesooders, Xhaoz, Agiseb, HamburgerRadio, Citation bot 1, Careful With That Axe, Eugene, Chenopodiaceous, Intelligentsium, Pinethicket, Elockid, Edderso, Abductive, KyleDude96, Joshuashua, Xxemiixx, Calmer Waters, Hamtechperson, Wikitza, A8UDI, Mellie.N.D, RedBot, SpaceFlight89, VinnyXY, Takmina, LLThom, Monkeymanman, Newgrounder, Carolina cotton, Merlion444, Jauhienij, Cookiesv, CovenantWord, Samuel Salzman, Abc518, EfAston, Kgrad, TrickyM, Champion97, Fesaitu, DriveMySol, Sheogorath, Comnenus, Pitcroft, Shiyu918, Lotje, TONIC WATER, VNNS, Gulbenk, Toniiiix, Epic Penguin123, TheMIH, Bingo1326, The-GrimReaper NS, Diannaa, DaDouche2, TwistedMidnight, Peacedance, Tbhotch, Brody6900, Reach Out to the Truth, Jarpup, DARTH SIDIOUS 2, Andrea105, Minicl55, RjwilmsiBot, 7mike5000, Acbistro, Regancy42, Hrvatistan, Agent Smith (The Matrix), Anthonybouzi, Salvio giuliano, Slon02, Toofox, LcawteHuggle, Bowei Huang, DASHBot, EmausBot, I:)Pie124578, Az29, Look2See1, Chickeral, Cvbbocvbbob, Qwertybutt, Hazzy Teh Nub, DotKuro, Daddy303dank, Loisandizzyrules, Mmoor15, People100, Qwertyrandom, John Cline, Bongoramsey, Schnauzendorf, Catalaalatac, DJ Tricky86, H3llBot, AndrewOne, AManWithNoPlan, Wayne Slam, Ocaasi, Shammy97, IGeMiNix, Brandmeister, Uspastpresentwatch2010, Superbrutaka07, Seriouslyshouldjustbe, Clementina, Herk1955, BetterInternet, Mikeytrousers, DASHBotAV, Seltzerfish, Dylando0, Timemaps, Grapple X, ClueBot NG, Anagoria, ⯑, 6ii9, A wild Rattata, Frietjes, Mesoderm, Lauren68, Helpful Pixie Bot, Newyork1501, Guest2625, Regulov, BG19bot, Theherald1000, Dutchldy, Eric567, JohnChrysostom, Zaltaire, User1961914, Cold Season, Tintaggon, AdventurousSquirrel, Yerevantsi, CitationCleanerBot, Harizotoh9, MrBill3, Polmandc, 220 of Borg, Mauramerck, ChrisGualtieri, Chafinsky, Khazar2, Illia Connell, Dexbot, Mogism, Jeccabreen, Brentwood Ontario, AldezD, Numancia, Gabelglesia, MarchOrDie, Cam04, Rachellains, Seraborum, Waddlesplash, Joncat123, Wethar555, Dairhead, CensoredScribe, IQ125, Spyglasses, Wyatt117halo, Kind Tennis Fan, Man of Steel 85, Moonchïld9, Monkbot, IAreC4, Nearwater, JasonWars, Skyb0x, Maltrópa, Sayekang, JamiePringle and Anonymous: 2691

- **Bubonic plague** *Source:* https://en.wikipedia.org/wiki/Bubonic_plague?oldid=688279110 *Contributors:* William Avery, Frecklefoot, Ubiquity, Ixfd64, Mdebets, Darkwind, Julesd, Jeandré du Toit, Topbanana, Phil Boswell, Sunray, Saforrest, Xanzzibar, DocWatson42, Everyking, Jackol, Kjetil r, OverlordQ, JulieADriver, Ukexpat, Dcandeto, Alperen, Mike Rosoft, Discospinster, Rich Farmbrough, Smyth, Bender235, Kbh3rd, Neko-chan, MBisanz, EmilJ, Arancaytar, Bobo192, Smalljim, Wisdom89, Angie Y., Arcadian, ParticleMan, Hajenso, Nsaa, Jakew, Storm Rider, Stephen G. Brown, Patsw, Alansohn, Guy Harris, Arthena, Supine, Andrewpmk, Wouterstomp, SlimVirgin, Bucephalus, Velella, TaintedMustard, Kdau, Amorymeltzer, RainbowOfLight, Sciurinæ, Blaxthos, Angr, Richard Arthur Norton (1958-), Mindmatrix, Camw, Nuggetboy, Scjessey, Zealander, JBellis, WadeSimMiser, MONGO, Kmg90, John Hill, Isnow, Kriegman, Prashanthns, Abd, Dysepsion, Graham87, WBardwin, BD2412, Abach, Mendaliv, Pmj, Rjwilmsi, Coemgenus, CyberGhostface, Jake Wartenberg, Bruce1ee, The wub, DoubleBlue, RobertG, Latka, Nihiltres, Gurch, President Rhapsody, TeaDrinker, Jaraalbe, Sharkface217, DVdm, Sceptre, Ste1n, Jimp, Kymacpherson, Damiangerous, Rsrikanth05, David R. Ingham, NawlinWiki, Grafen, Erielhonan, ZacBowling, Rjensen, Dogcow, Brian Crawford, Moe Epsilon, Syrthiss, Rwalker, Barnabypage, Brisvegas, Werdna, Wknight94, Daniel C, Newagelink, Aremisasling, Closedmouth, Nkendrick, Red Jay, CWenger, Katieh5584, TLSuda, ChemGardener, SmackBot, Unschool, Espresso Addict, Cubs Fan, PAR1138, C.Fred, Jab843, Gilliam, Hmains, Skizzik, Persian Poet Gal, Jprg1966, Deli nk, Darth Panda, Rizzardi, Gsp8181, Muboshgu, Onorem, Lennylim, Kcordina, Decltype, Jwy, VegaDark, Acdx, Bejnar, Risssa, Drunken Pirate, Zaxius, Kuru, John, Mwanafunzi~enwiki, Aleenf1, Physis, Yogesh Khandke, A. Parrot, Soulkeeper, BillFlis, Stwalkerster, Davemcarlson, Boomshadow, Sinistrum, Larrymcp, Waggers, Me2NiK, Citicat, Norm mit, Iridescent, Rainbow Warrior, Twas Now, KsprayDad, Igoldste, CapitalR, Courcelles, Boucher4, Chovain, Chris55, FatalError, J Milburn, JForget, Liam Skoda, Unionhawk, ArmyOfFluoride, Rwflammang, Cocomonkilla, Ruslik0, ShelfSkewed, Stevv, Xylir, Funnyfarmofdoom, Themightyquill, Cydebot, Ryan, Reywas92, Grahamec, Mato, Vanished user vjhsduheuiui4t5hjri, Gogo Dodo, Anthonyhcole, Markwpage, Shirulashem, FDV, Agnostoman, SpK, Myhlow, Vanished User jdksfajlasd, Zalgo, Realdog, Citizen6ix, Thijs!bot, Epbr123, Qwyrxian, Jmg38, HappyInGeneral, N5iln, Oliver202, Marek69, Itsmejudith, CTZMSC3, PottersWood, Escarbot, Seaphoto, Cbrucker, QuiteUnusual, Doc Tropics, VectorPosse, Shadow girl, LibLord, Kaini, Gökhan, Res2216firestar, JAnDbot, Xhienne, D99figge, Leuko, Matthew Fennell, Awien, Flying tiger, Connormah, Pedro, Bongwarrior, VoABot II, Jonwillig, AuburnPilot, AtticusX, Fbdave, Doug Coldwell, Whisk3rs, Tedickey, Nyttend, Avicennasis, WhatamIdoing, Dorte Nielsen, ForestAngel, 28421u2232nfenfcenc, Cpl Syx, Debollweevil, JaGa, Philg88, Tapioca Dextrin, Karengpve, Angelo Somaschini, FisherQueen, Turiyag, NAHID, MaraNeo127, AlexiusHoratius, Ash, EdBever, Tgeairn, Dinkytown, AlphaEta, J.delanoy, Pharaoh of the Wizards, Nev1, Trusilver, Entre5et7, Bogey97, Uncle Dick, Headinthedoor, Ginsengbomb, Gorndog, Icseaturtles, Shawn in Montreal, Katalaveno, Warmwasser, WebHamster, (jarbarf), LA Songs, Aznsamurai11, NewEnglandYankee, Molly-in-md, SJP, Ferahgo the Assassin, Ionescuac, Juliancolton, Adamd1008, Vanished user 39948282, Devmoz, Pdcook, Ja 62, Useight, CardinalDan, Funandtrvl, Wikieditor06, My Core Competency is Competency, Deor, Hammersoft, CWii, ABF, Jeff G., Indubitably, Bacchus87, Satani, VasilievVV, Ryan032, DelphinusMach1, Philip Trueman, Cosmic Latte, GcSwRhIc, Monkey Bounce, Piperh, Oxfordwang, Martin451, Jackfork, Amog, Optigan13, Slimfan3, Rumiton, Blurpeace, Ximodnic, Meters, Synthebot, Falcon8765, Enviroboy, JukoFF, Petethebloke, Brianga, Monty845, Chenzw, Doc James, Mikemoral, Sonicology, Tresiden, Jauerback, Jaeran, Winchelsea, YourEyesOnly, Dawn Bard, 1337pino, Logarkh, Interchange88, Bentogoa, Flyer22 Reborn, Prestonmag, Mimihitam, Antonio Lopez, PhilMacD, Bagatelle, Tombomp, Archaeogenetics, Techman224, Joshii, WacoJacko, Ctxppc, StaticGull, Realm of Shadows, Dimboukas, Nn123645, H1nkles, Escape Orbit, Kanonkas, Explicit, Mr. Granger, Atif.t2, Loren.wilton, Albert Krantz, De728631, ClueBot, GorillaWarfare, Marydell, Fyyer, Kotniski, The Thing That Should Not Be, Ndenison, R000t, Arakunem, Shinpah1, Uncle Milty, SuperHamster, Boing! said Zebedee, Awesomemccoy18, Blanchardb, Parkwells, Piledhigheranddeeper, Neverquick, Arunsingh16, Publius Publicola, Excirial, Jusdafax, Dr.orfannkyl, Emuland, Tyler, Tacoman2, Arjayay, Sbfw, K-Billy~enwiki, Yizhenwilliam, CowboySpartan, Fattyjwoods, BOTarate, Thehelpfulone, Bald Zebra, Catalographer, Thingg, Aitias, DerBorg, Subash.chandran007, Versus22, Crowsnest, Chloer7600, Templarion, BendersGame, BarretB, Against the current, XLinkBot, BodhisattvaBot, Rror, Dthomsen8, Nepenthes, Little Mountain 5, Facts707, Kytsday, NellieBly, Lvova, Alexius08, Noctibus, Gazimoff, Sjdist2012, TravisAF, ZooFari, MagnesianPhoenix, Catgirl, Good Olfactory, Airplaneman, By Little Old Me, RyanCross, Addbot, Willking1979, Some jerk on the Internet, Whirling within, Jojhutton, Scientamata, Atethnekos, DougsTech, Prairieplant, 15lsoucy, Ronhjones, Hellokitty7484, Fieldday-sunday, Mr. Wheely Guy, Underwaterbuffalo, CanadianLinuxUser, Leszek Jańczuk, Captainlanks, Cst17, SoSaysChappy, Morning277, Chamal N, Ld100, Debresser, XRK, Doniago, Lucian Sunday, LinkFA-Bot, Tatesgay, Tyw7, Batamt, KaiKemmann, Terrillja, Meaters2, Tide rolls, Bfigura's puppy, Jan eissfeldt, Y.B, זרות55, Jamie naik, Genius101, Doodlydoo, Frehley, Swusr, Luckas-bot, Dillardjj, Yobot, Legolas173, Fraggle81, Legobot II, Newportm, Terrifictriffid, PM-Lawrence, Lfc4lyf08, THEN WHO WAS PHONE?, SwisterTwister, IW.HG, Tempodivalse, Backslash Forwardslash, AnomieBOT, KDS4444, Wikieditoroftoday, Oxford pictionary, Hairhorn, Marauder40, Kristen Eriksen, Coopkev2, Slaterino, Jim1138, Pyrrhus16, Piano non troppo, Aditya, Ninahexan, Kingpin13, Ulric1313, Flewis, Ckruschke, The High Fin Sperm Whale, Danno uk, Citation bot, Calmer Llama, E2eamon, Jock Boy, Maxis ftw, Nealvince, GB fan, ChristianH, Xqbot, Jay77710, Cureden, Strykerblade, Mch007, Addihockey10, Capricorn42, Drilnoth, 4twenty42o, Nasnema, Stars4change, Jsharpminor, Grim23, The Evil IP address, Tyrol5, Inferno, Lord of Penguins, Ableadded, Briony Coote, Abce2, AlecStewart, Brandon5485, SassoBot, Bellerophon, Wnme, Mathonius, Amaury, Arturkjakub, Brutaldeluxe, Hellomovie, Doulos Christos, Drdpw, N419BH, Smallman12q, Natural Cut, Crw9961, In fact, Shadowjams, WaysToEscape, Chanzec1, Erik9, Mjasfca, A.amitkumar, Dougofborg, Celuici, Lolipop101, FrescoBot, Surv1v4l1st, Pepper, Tophee1, Oldlaptop321, Heads963, RicHard-59, SMOKEMOREPOT, Peachezinurmouth, Elsie33, Nigelgenders, Oashi, Sxhpb, Nimbulus00, Citation bot 1, Ntse, Slobodan Grasic, DrilBot, Eagles13 13, Cesue, Pinethicket, I dream of horses, Abductive, Spandumb, Temple mara, PrincessofLlyr, 10metreh, Calmer Waters, A8UDI, Magical Mayhem 007, BRUTE, ContinueWithCaution, Île flottante, Жељко Тодоровић, SlipknotRlZZ, Utility Monster, PerV, Skwirel, Bayxsonic, Thomasmitchell666, Trappist the monk, Sheogorath, Jonkerz, Lotje, Obbly1, BlackAce48, Mrgagafoo, Vrenator, TBloemink, Clarkcj12, JumpDiscont, Stegop, Jem54, Diannaa, Weedwhacker128, Clrbear430, Tbhotch, Brody6900, Scatman160, Reach Out to the Truth, Bongdentoiac, Daniel the Monk, Sideways713, Typarkison, DARTH SIDIOUS 2, Jfmantis, Greghhepburn, Mindy Dirt, RjwilmsiBot, 7mike5000, Hyarmendacil, Björn-Bergman, Woovee, Pigwhopoopscats, Salvio giuliano, Kiko4564, Deagle AP, DASHBot, Esoglou, J36miles, EmausBot, Oliverlyc, SkyeSlaughter, Acather96, Immunize, Gfoley4, Sophie, ECTaiwan2010, Hobbesss, Racerx11, Kkk888, GoingBatty, RA0808, Eruditegirl, Dishcmds, Finn Bjørklid, Slightsmile, Tommy2010, Lokithetroublemaker, Kidcozy, Wikipelli, Choosebrad, Thecheesykid, Savh, Ckramar18, Weathergossip, John Cline, Érico, Wackywace, Eyadhamid, EWikist, SporkBot, Netha Hussain, Tolly4bolly, Cmathio, Connor444424, Jsayre64, Arman Cagle, Coasterlover1994, Michaelallenonline, L Kensington, Donner60, Puffin, Judygreenberg, Spacehunny, Orange Suede Sofa, Gunbound4234, DASHBotAV, Spicemix, ClueBot NG, Gareth Griffith-Jones, Awkwardspam, Emikate518, Satellizer, Samgoinham, Johnsmith10111994, Highestdood, Diabalo17, Seanypoo123, Delusion23, Evanc1310, Ap27627, Adwiii, Widr, Antiqueight, Asdfjkl1234, SuperCoder, Planet SIC, MerllwBot, Helpful Pixie Bot, Burritoman123456, Otmp, Ryannm123, Nightenbelle, Ryannm1234, DBigXray, Guest2625, Bassikj, Lowercase sigmabot, Hurling dervish, Dutch54, Kenfreak, EvilResident, WikiTryHardDieHard, Footballrules123, Radovan lipic 1999, Idfviudfivuhdifu-vhdfjbn, Ecimino, Tayye.briannon12, Who.was.phone, MusikAnimal, Mark Arsten, AdventurousSquirrel, Altaïr, Harizotoh9, Snow Blizzard, MrBill3, Jaciek, Glacialfox, Jodie25, Worldiswatching, Snu7, Galbano, Klilidiplomus, Langenberg at Central College, Xomusicxo9, Natrunman, Haitchnash, Nascraytia, EricEnfermero, BattyBot, Reedy1871, Lukas²³, Liam987, Master91702, FatFace1, Th4n3r, DemirBajraktarevic, Ushau97, ChrisGualtieri, Cwcm98, JesseAlanGordon, Leah17kiss, Dexbot, Jpcivin, Brass razoo, Zeeyanwiki, FoCuSandLeArN, Jboogy25, Mogism, Skyrimnerdgirl, Lugia2453, Buffalonuts, John.allison.2, Molenchuk, Corn cheese, JustAMuggle, Gabenewll, Epicgenius, Chihuahua-hater411, Theteekel, Usernamehere90840, ChryslerChrome, 14bylerkasey, JPaestpreornJeolhlna, Biomedicinal, Stickman1270, Swagmeout999, NLMOCPL, Coolne, DavidLeighEllis, TurtleTom1096, Anime Batman, Matt.erney, Taytothta56, Darkknight4230, Ginsuloft, Markieeedark-ieee, Sam Sailor, NicNacAttack, Princesslyons, Asfasfashfuitdfgisd, Westingc, Cyu7, Riddleh, Monkbot, Gunnar3281, FutureMan America and Anonymous: 1478

- **Dalhana** *Source:* https://en.wikipedia.org/wiki/Dalhana?oldid=635991584 *Contributors:* Dbachmann, Jodosma and Bladesmulti

- **Hakim Syed Zillur Rahman** *Source:* https://en.wikipedia.org/wiki/Hakim_Syed_Zillur_Rahman?oldid=685155734 *Contributors:* Jossi, Rich Farmbrough, Woohookitty, Kosher Fan, Jaraalbe, Wavelength, Anomie, Welsh, Tsalman, Tachs, SmackBot, Spasage, Betacommand, Wizard-man, Ohconfucius, Shyamsunder, Cydebot, BetacommandBot, Rzafar, RobotG, IndianGeneralist, Ekabhishek, Faizhaider, Waacstats, JaGa, Szrahman, EmanWilm, Muhandes, SchreiberBike, Addbot, Yobot, Gongshow, AnomieBOT, LilHelpa, Gilo1969, Erik9bot, LittleWink, Bg-paulus, GoingBatty, Ibnsinaacademy, Hashemi1971, Mar4d, Jschauhan, Ramansoz, Vacation9, Helpful Pixie Bot, Shaad lko, Mitchitara, Jawad physics, Spiderjerky, KasparBot and Anonymous: 12

- **Ibn Sina Academy of Medieval Medicine and Sciences** *Source:* https://en.wikipedia.org/wiki/Ibn_Sina_Academy_of_Medieval_Medicine_and_Sciences?oldid=690099543 *Contributors:* Bearcat, Varlaam, Woohookitty, Lmatt, RussBot, Dialectric, Jpbowen, Tsalman, Bazonka, Shyamsunder, Imransabri, Dr Greg, Cydebot, Ekabhishek, JamesBWatson, Jllm06, JaGa, DGG, R'n'B, Naniwako, Roland zh, Szrahman, Icarusgeek, Muhandes, Ironholds, Chzz, Tassedethe, Yobot, FrescoBot, Kajervi, Hashemi1971, Midas02, Jschauhan, Ramansoz, Crown Prince, DR.ABDUL LATIF, Way2veers and Anonymous: 6

- **Jarrah (Surgeon)** *Source:* https://en.wikipedia.org/wiki/Jarrah_(Surgeon)?oldid=568976905 *Contributors:* Asarelah, Shyamsunder, NewEng-landYankee, FrescoBot, RjwilmsiBot, John of Reading, Omer123hussain, RotlinkBot, Evano1van and Anonymous: 1

- **Lapidary (text)** *Source:* https://en.wikipedia.org/wiki/Lapidary_(text)?oldid=585470289 *Contributors:* Wavelength, Nikkimaria, R'n'B, John-bod and DoctorKubla

- **Leper colony** *Source:* https://en.wikipedia.org/wiki/Leper_colony?oldid=686428694 *Contributors:* DopefishJustin, Bueller 007, Andres, Jen-god, Choster, Bhs, Maximus Rex, Scott Sanchez, Pakaran, Gentgeen, Robbot, Meelar, Robartin, PBP, Triptych, Alan Liefting, Comatose51, Mackeriv, Mschlindwein, Vapour, Notinasnaid, Guettarda, Deathawk, Jonathunder, Jumbuck, Richard Harvey, MarkRose, StJarvitude, Ste-monitis, AirBa~enwiki, MarcoTolo, Graham87, Rjwilmsi, Hathawayc, Spasemunki, Vmenkov, Jpfagerback, YurikBot, Splash, Kimchi.sg, Michalis Famelis, Unforgiven24, Eaefremov, Demogorgon's Soup-taster, Anonimu, SmackBot, AeternNull, Mihail ioniu~enwiki, Gilliam, Al-gont, Jxm, Swat671, Bigturtle, Thegraham, Kukini, Stewie814, LFenske, Peyre, Iridescent, Joseph Solis in Australia, Mattbr, Aherunar, Aza-kreski, Themightyquill, Phenss, Michaelas10, Mubariz, Racaille, Missvain, Escarbot, Golf Bravo, Dougher, Ingolfson, Gramjoy777, Magi-oladitis, Superjoo, Nyttend, Migp, 28421u2232nfenfcenc, MartinBot, BeadleB, UBeR, Piercetheorganist, MsgrCloche, Johnbod, Naniwako, Totoro-chan, ACSE, Polarbear97, Philip Trueman, R45, YangYouRen, Erobinson30, Staveley, ClueBot, Piledhigheranddeeper, Catalographer, 1Temp, DumZiBoT, Ridemate, XLinkBot, Pogo-Pogo-Pogo, Addbot, LaaknorBot, Morning277, Ld100, Tide rolls, Lightbot, Rubinbot, Tech-Bot, FrescoBot, Shanghainese.ua, Kgrad, Ichiro Kikuchi, ClueBot NG, Primergrey, Widr, Compfreak7, Rococo1700, Cyberbot II, ElŞahin, Kohelet, Lsavassi, KasparBot, OrganicEarth and Anonymous: 99

- **MacDunleavy/MacNulty physicians of Tirconnell** *Source:* https://en.wikipedia.org/wiki/MacDunleavy/MacNulty_physicians_of_Tirconnell?oldid=634546778 *Contributors:* Ohconfucius, Funandtrvl, Yobot, Aisteco, Albiet and Anonymous: 1

- **Matthaeus Silvaticus** *Source:* https://en.wikipedia.org/wiki/Matthaeus_Silvaticus?oldid=659379474 *Contributors:* GTBacchus, Mervyn, FeanorStar7, Canadian Paul, Rjwilmsi, Chris the speller, Missvain, Seanwal111111, Addbot, RjwilmsiBot, Ripchip Bot, Djembayz, Chuis-pastonBot and KasparBot

- **Plague doctor** *Source:* https://en.wikipedia.org/wiki/Plague_doctor?oldid=689353769 *Contributors:* SimonP, Tzaquiel, Charles Matthews, Di-madick, Timrollpickering, Xanzzibar, Christopher Parham, Yugure, Fergananim, DNewhall, Discospinster, Kbh3rd, CanisRufus, Wareh, Cour-tarro, Nkedel, Hq3473, NantonosAedui, Woohookitty, ApLundell, Nightscream, Rtkat3, Grafen, Krea, Moe Epsilon, Zackarotto, Kortoso, Asarelah, SmackBot, McGeddon, Gilliam, Skizzik, Chris the speller, Ikiroid, Esprix, Egsan Bacon, Valenciano, Ian Spackman, Mon Vier, A. Parrot, Vagary, Killer ninjas, IdiotSavant, Shandris, Edwardx, Handface, Soimless, Doug Coldwell, CommonsDelinker, PapalAuthoritah, AlphaEta, Philip Trueman, Burpen, Andrewaskew, Michaeldsuarez, SieBot, Dawn Bard, Flyer22 Reborn, Sean.hoyland, Excirial, Rhododen-drites, 7&6=thirteen, Avoided, MystBot, Osarius, Felix Folio Secundus, Addbot, Lolsimon, Non-dropframe, AttoRenato, Download, Tide rolls, Math Champion, Luckas-bot, MileyDavidA, AnomieBOT, KDS4444, Materialscientist, JimVC3, NFD9001, PimRijkee, Mathonius, Celuici, Lotje, Vrenator, TBloemink, Aoidh, Pruis, EmausBot, WikitanvirBot, Mikemacdee, SidoniaBorcke, ZéroBot, Josve05a, A930913, Donner60, Carmichael, ChuispastonBot, ClueBot NG, Jack Greenmaven, Satellizer, Lord Roem, Widr, Helpful Pixie Bot, WNYY98, Sergei RND, Mitchi-tara, Klilidiplomus, EagerToddler39, Hmainsbot1, Teleohapsis, Frosty, Thunderchief97, NZVortex, Wywin, Bugzeeolboy, Epicgenius, Lizy7, Hi Phi Pi, Tentinator, Ahov, ElHef, Mgrantham18, Eric Corbett, Gomotlopgo, Supertregamer, BethNaught, Lolage32121, Zacwill, Mad-man123467, Asdklf;, KH-1, ScarfaceGP1234, Supdiop, Turtle Fatality, Bobbyleponge and Anonymous: 165

- **Studies of the Fetus in the Womb** *Source:* https://en.wikipedia.org/wiki/Studies_of_the_Fetus_in_the_Womb?oldid=674959054 *Contributors:* Brandmeister and BG19bot

- **Unani medicine** *Source:* https://en.wikipedia.org/wiki/Unani_medicine?oldid=690276389 *Contributors:* SimonP, Olivier, Leandrod, Ronz, Justin Bacon, Topbanana, Dimadick, Phil Boswell, Diderot, SWAdair, Utcursch, Mozzerati, Discospinster, Dbachmann, ESkog, Kwamik-agami, Giraffedata, Idleguy, Ish ishwar, P Ingerson, Mahanga, Angr, John Gohde, SDC, SeventyThree, Graham87, Xenoncloud, BD2412, Rjwilmsi, Smithfarm, AED, Hmonroe, Random user 39849958, Wavelength, Waitak, RussBot, DanMS, Dialectric, Welsh, Shahcts, BirgitteSB, Lockesdonkey, Muzammil786, Jpeob, 2over0, JoanneB, SmackBot, Slashme, Jagged 85, Apers0n, Mairibot, Bluebot, Hibernian, Deli nk,

Downwards, Ne0Freedom, BullRangifer, Bahauddeen, Raabbasi, NandaAbeysekera, Shyamsunder, Lapiseyed, AlmightyDoctor, Arkrishna, Jason7825, Hebrides, Adri K., Trengarasu, Scientizzle fo bizzle, C56C, Deflective, Ekabhishek, Alt f in, Drasad, JNW, Kajasudhakarababu, Habib v, WhatamIdoing, Ian.thomson, Naniwako, Nadiatalent, Geekdiva, Signalhead, Technopat, Eubulides, Kashif72, Dr N D King, JamesStewart7, J8079s, Doseiai2, JTSchreiber, SchreiberBike, Yozer1, XLinkBot, Staticshakedown, Kavish555in, Dthomsen8, Shoemaker's Holiday, Addbot, Power.corrupts, Verbal, Lightbot, Anees345, Luckas-bot, Yobot, Ptbotgourou, Fraggle81, AR Thomson, AnomieBOT, AmritasyaPutra, Khadijah34, Xqbot, Nasnema, J04n, Momomatic, FrescoBot, Energyworm, Avijjan, SweetGeek2, RedBot, Drasadpasha, 564dude, Tbhotch, RjwilmsiBot, Look2See1, Dewritech, ZxxZxxZ, Solarra, ZéroBot, Hashemi1971, Mar4d, Ss charley, Davormax, Walkerville01, Ramansoz, ClueBot NG, Dream of Nyx, Widr, Helpful Pixie Bot, Draminaifrtk, Curb Chain, Hkmarahman, Shaad Iko, Muqueem4040, Sumaiya snigdha, PhnomPencil, Davidiad, CitationCleanerBot, Uzma.manzar, ChrisGualtieri, Dexbot, Jockzain, SantoshBot, Hotmuru, Drkashifalig, Pankaj Oudhia, UsmanullahPK, Uzairbaqai, Bladesmulti, Nannadeem, Dehlvimohsin, Monkbot, ☐☐☐☐Hakim dr rais khan, Happiest persoN, Awamilabs, Profansarizaki, Vreswiki, Projecthashmi, Mheydari2, Sadrifoundation, Hamidone, MirHaiderAli and Anonymous: 117

- **Unicorn horn** *Source:* https://en.wikipedia.org/wiki/Unicorn_horn?oldid=681885637 *Contributors:* Xanzzibar, Furius, JSH-alive, Bongwarrior, JamesBWatson, Cnilep, EoGuy, Drmies, Niceguyedc, Addbot, Yobot, Andreasmperu, Materialscientist, Pinethicket, Kelly2357, John of Reading, Robin Lionheart, The White Hart of Wikiwood, ClueBot NG, TornadoLGS, Dexbot, Hmainsbot1, Xenxax, Monkbot, Jayakumar RG, Taterthottttttt69 and Anonymous: 17

- **Bimaristan** *Source:* https://en.wikipedia.org/wiki/Bimaristan?oldid=681434756 *Contributors:* Cimon Avaro, Antandrus, Neutrality, Ogress, Alansohn, Jheald, Rjwilmsi, Angusmclellan, Koavf, Srleffler, Imnotminkus, NawlinWiki, Dialectric, Trovatore, SmackBot, Jagged 85, ParthianShot, Chris the speller, Avin, Cloj, Colonies Chris, Jmlk17, John, Cydebot, Mato, Mattisse, DuncanHill, Rich257, الدبوني, Gun Powder Ma, Stephenchou0722, R'n'B, Pharaoh of the Wizards, Crystalu, Ctesiphon7, Intothefire, SamuelTheGhost, Ashashyou, CohesionBot, Al-Andalusi, Joe N, Addbot, DOI bot, Tassedethe, Luckas-bot, Yobot, AnomieBOT, Citation bot, Jtamad, Fatepur, FrescoBot, Citation bot 1, Lotje, على ویکی, Syncategoremata, ZxxZxxZ, AvicBot, Jesanj, L Kensington, Helpful Pixie Bot, Yamaha5, YiFeiBot and Anonymous: 9

- **Byzantine medicine** *Source:* https://en.wikipedia.org/wiki/Byzantine_medicine?oldid=659962100 *Contributors:* Llywrch, Adam Bishop, Wetman, Sjorford, Tom harrison, Varlaam, Macrakis, Kuralyov, Stbalbach, Firsfron, NickOfCyprus, GreekWarrior, SmackBot, Jagged 85, Betacommand, Bluebot, Cplakidas, CmdrObot, Mukake, Ujalm, VolkovBot, Butterscotch, J8079s, Doseiai2, Addbot, Atethnekos, SpBot, Lightbot, Yobot, Ptbotgourou, Kibi78704, Correctionwriter, ClueBot NG, Helpful Pixie Bot, Smeat75, Pseudoneiros, Torvalu4, Mogism, AndyHarwell, Leedlepoo107, Funfeat, Ugog Nizdast, Sairp and Anonymous: 15

- **Cupping therapy** *Source:* https://en.wikipedia.org/wiki/Cupping_therapy?oldid=690734972 *Contributors:* Hyacinth, Phoebe, Bearcat, Postdlf, SchmuckyTheCat, Walloon, David Gerard, Vasi, Art Carlson, Ferdinand Pienaar, Bosmon, Lacrimosus, Discospinster, Rich Farmbrough, LeeHunter, Elwikipedista~enwiki, Femto, Wee Jimmy, Roganhamby, Alansohn, Aliparsa, Cypherpunk, Bart133, Fourthords, Danaman5, Garzo, Goulo, PatGallacher, Alanmak, WadeSimMiser, GregorB, Graham87, Rjwilmsi, Nightscream, Bensin, Maurog, JdforresterBot, RexNL, Gurch, Jrtayloriv, Travis.Thurston, YurikBot, Rabid Hamster, Shell Kinney, CambridgeBayWeather, Dialectric, Badagnani, Mccready, Tearlach, Malcolma, Matticus78, SM, Procedure, Asarelah, 2over0, Cspalletta, Tevildo, NetRolller 3D, SmackBot, PiCo, Sticky Parkin, Shai-kun, Gilliam, Deli nk, Nbarth, Frap, Шизомби, George, BullRangifer, Politis, Rigadoun, Raoodee, Salmanjafri, IronGargoyle, Meco, Iridescent, Skapur, StephenBuxton, Ewulp, Kbarends, Eikaj, CuriousEric, Pointedstick, Mato, Lindsay658, Dianelowe, Midnight coffee, Thijs!bot, Angievirus, Mojo Hand, I do not exist, AntiVandalBot, Magioladitis, Drasad, Soulbot, Fcjohn, KConWiki, WLU, Ghorbanalibeik, AstroHurricane001, MistyMorn, OohBunnies!, Geekdiva, Rewayah, Funandtrvl, Sam Blacketer, VolkovBot, Attilio74, AlnoktaBOT, TXiKiBoT, Chisource, Spiral5800, Falcon8765, Centerone, Ttony21, Flyer22 Reborn, Alexbrn, Theroyalweman, Pharmtao, Bentevb, ClueBot, Brokenearth, EoGuy, Drmies, Qsaw, Niceguyedc, Pakistan Tiger, Excirial, Alexbot, Signpostmaker, M.O.X, The Red, Al-Andalusi, Nakomaru, Graham1973, Apparition11, Acuhealth, Mr. Gerbear, Drbilals, Addbot, Mouäwen, DOI bot, Queenmomcat, Ocdnctx, Mootros, Leszek Jańczuk, Tsange, Tassedethe, Tide rolls, Teles, Zorrobot, Lukasz2, Legobot, Luckas-bot, Yobot, Ptbotgourou, AnomieBOT, JaneSchmo, Smcauley, Sz-iwbot, Tamershaban, DSisyphBot, Anna Frodesiak, Signpost64, RibotBOT, Mastermariox, Chkwiki, فيصل الحويطي, FrescoBot, Jusses2, Blesstheusa, Vrenator, CleverTitania, Beyond My Ken, Musenett, Rayman60, WikitanvirBot, Chelos, ScottyBerg, RA0808, Solarra, Ahmed899, ZéroBot, Jenks24, A930913, Jhcapps, BeNothing, SBaker43, Txus.aparicio, Brother Bulldog, 28bot, Manytexts, Helpsome, ClueBot NG, Sakudesu, This lousy T-shirt, Cntras, Curb Chain, BG19bot, Island Monkey, DerrickZ, Kalsession1892, Hamahardi, Realize This, BrokenEarthOrg, Dean bosley, Cctvna, Project Osprey, Ericcartmanfat, Margirl1459, Ahaiahai, Epicgenius, Ruby Murray, Lowkeyvision, Everymorning, Scarabola, Jpsanders, Ninjaalga, Davidfang2000, Louieunfitz, Monkbot, Gormadoc, Efrances93, Karinpower, Cgq144, Helenead, EJAZ RANA, Lac907, Lilyhuegerich, Nathealth123, Nieuwzeelander, 1928Whippet, Shajeda and Anonymous: 217

- **Dodecapharmacum** *Source:* https://en.wikipedia.org/wiki/Dodecapharmacum?oldid=574224141 *Contributors:* Yobot, Gråbergs Gråa Sång, In ictu oculi, John of Reading, Mogism and Drali1954

- **Exorcism in Islam** *Source:* https://en.wikipedia.org/wiki/Exorcism_in_Islam?oldid=665662236 *Contributors:* Mr. Granger, Al-Andalusi, Addbot, WikiDan61, Asif756, ClueBot NG, Umairdr82, Chintu6, GoodParabolē, DrRNC, Jackmcbarn, Admiral Caius, Shafi (Abdalshafi) Ghwerien, يماني and Anonymous: 8

- **Hijama** *Source:* https://en.wikipedia.org/wiki/Hijama?oldid=688072832 *Contributors:* SchmuckyTheCat, Jason Quinn, Chowbok, Sonjaaa, Pearle, Javidan, Bobrayner, Ruud Koot, Rjwilmsi, Koavf, Bgwhite, CambridgeBayWeather, Eleassar, Tearlach, Bobak, Froth, Asarelah, A13ean, SmackBot, Sticky Parkin, Sigma 7, Mcshadypl, Robofish, IronGargoyle, Meco, IvanLanin, CmdrObot, Cydebot, Mercury~enwiki, GLGerman~enwiki, Makerowner, Ichibani, AA, MelkorDCLXVI, Jubrankhalil, SieBot, Monsort, Iwansw, Mohummy, Ultrabias, Brokenearth, Supertouch, Signpostmaker, Al-Andalusi, Aitias, Tomyarbro, Yozer1, XLinkBot, Hotcrocodile, Ali Esfandiari, Salam32, Addbot, Folatib, Micahmedia, Legobot, Yobot, AnomieBOT, Arjun G. Menon, Materialscientist, Xqbot, Bihco, Signpost64, Njod, Chkwiki, FrescoBot, Achaemenes, Tbhotch, TjBot, John of Reading, Trilliumz, RA0808, SporkBot, BeNothing, SBaker43, ClueBot NG, Widr, Ramaksoud2000, Mod1101, Curiouscattoo, Pratyya Ghosh, HacksBack, BrokenEarthOrg, Saedon, Cerabot~enwiki, Ericcartmanfat, Passengerpigeon, Lowkeyvision, Drmoiniidd, UmarRab, YiFeiBot, Ibensis, Hijama Clinic Sunnah, Aminealoulou82, Sharif uddin, Quantum.Ruqya, Yousef Qassem, Hijama, Pbuhmedicine, Granada12, Raynee.j, Yasskand and Anonymous: 73

- **Medicine in the medieval Islamic world** *Source:* https://en.wikipedia.org/wiki/Medicine_in_the_medieval_Islamic_world?oldid=690649839 *Contributors:* William Avery, William M. Connolley, Julesd, Scott, Andrewman327, WhisperToMe, Cercamon, Timrollpickering, Orpheus, Neutrality, Adashiel, Discospinster, Rich Farmbrough, Dbachmann, Bender235, Kwamikagami, Bobo192, Physicistjedi, Flammifer, Famousdog, MPerel, Irishpunktom, ABCD, Jheald, Geraldshields11, Zereshk, Woohookitty, Mindmatrix, Merlinme, Daniel Case, Guy M, Ruud Koot,

Tabletop, Gil-Galad, Striver, BD2412, Kbdank71, Rjwilmsi, Angusmclellan, Koavf, Reinis, FayssalF, Ian Pitchford, Riddleme, Gwernol, Uk-Paolo, RussBot, Porturology, Anonymous editor, Pigman, Gaius Cornelius, NawlinWiki, Dialectric, Lowe4091, Bloodofox, Rjensen, Equilibrial, Brandon, Gadget850, DeadEyeArrow, Wujastyk, Doncram, Elkman, Wiqi55, Reyk, Pablo2garcia~enwiki, Cartwarmark, JLaTondre, SmackBot, WilyD, Jagged 85, Delldot, Aksi great, Gilliam, Ohnoitsjamie, Hmains, ParthianShot, Chris the speller, Keegan, Colonies Chris, Arab Hafez, RandomP, Wizardman, Salamurai, Ohconfucius, Tktktk, Mitso Bel, Afadel, Thom85, Tofoo, Tawkerbot2, Daedalus969, Tanthalas39, Halimah-bintdavid, ShelfSkewed, FlyingToaster, Casper2k3, Neelix, Hemlock Martinis, Cydebot, Ryan, Dadofsam, Anthonyhcole, Dancter, Shirulashem, SteveMcCluskey, Crum375, Krylonblue83, Barticus88, Missvain, AntiVandalBot, DuncanHill, Dsp13, Hut 8.5, Yahel Guhan, Ma000055, VoABot II, ‎باسم, Andy mci, Belgrade18, David Eppstein, Beagel, Gun Powder Ma, Kkrystian, MartinBot, R'n'B, CommonsDelinker, Nono64, Lamaybe, J.delanoy, Maurice Carbonaro, LordAnubisBOT, Belovedfreak, Squids and Chips, Medicineman84, Signalhead, Meiskam, VolkovBot, Philip Trueman, Thegingerninja, Crohnie, LOTRrules, Barkeep, Bballstud10, WRK, Wilson44691, OKBot, Mohummy, Jobas, Explicit, ImageRemovalBot, Athenean, ClueBot, PipepBot, The Thing That Should Not Be, Brokenearth, Plastikspork, Witchwooder, VQuakr, Mild Bill Hiccup, J8079s, Lantay77, Doseiai2, CounterVandalismBot, Poolback, Veraisme, Neverquick, SamuelTheGhost, Ashashyou, CohesionBot, HssanKachal, ChrisHodgesUK, Al-Andalusi, Thingg, Versus22, MelonBot, Johnuniq, SoxBot III, Xiquet, Roxy the dog, EastTN, Dthomsen8, WikiHead, MEDISLAR, Nicolae Coman, Kefi~enwiki, UnknownForEver, Addbot, DOI bot, Cathcart5, Alexander Bakunin, Ccacsmss, De-bresser, Tassedethe, Tide rolls, Verbal, Lightbot, Krano, ‎انی م, ‎⁇⁇⁇, Ben Ben, Luckas-bot, Yobot, Ptbotgourou, Gobbleswoggler, AnomieBOT, Materialscientist, Citation bot, LilHelpa, Carturo222, Poetaris, TechBot, Johnson5 jr., Wickedrob, Storyof, GrouchoBot, Twirligig, Jezhotwells, lop7789, Esfandieasil, Taryakii, Citation bot 1, Abductive, Fuzbaby, Jonesey95, RedBot, Sahar N Saleem, Piandcompany, Ozhistory, Meamwye, Trappist the monk, RjwilmsiBot, Misconceptions2, Msin10, In ictu oculi, Slon02, EmausBot, Dolescum, Immunize, Craxyxarc, Look2See1, Fly by Night, Syncategoremata, GoingBatty, Aquib American Muslim, K6ka, Djembayz, Hhaaf000, Knight1993, Aeonx, Snaevar, Someone65, Openstrings, BeNothing, Orange Suede Sofa, ChuispastonBot, Tentontunic, ClueBot NG, Jack Greenmaven, ScottSteiner, Helpful Pixie Bot, MusikAnimal, King of things98, Krisrich, AdventurousSquirrel, Lbeaulieu1, Kcollins11, Kbeisaw, Bissonar, Eamodeo, Harizotoh9, Lorien-drew, BattyBot, StarryGrandma, SkepticalRaptor, Daisyoopsy, Dexbot, Mogism, Jah Akins, FrigidNinja, HistoryofIran, Tentinator, Babitaarora, Ugog Nizdast, Jbanerdt, HDSKhan, Ginsuloft, Jackmcbarn, JaconaFrere, BITYVITY, Yvetal, Gani94, Monkbot, Vieque, Evyslwyn, Mhhossein, ChloeDarke, Crazynyancat, Amortias, 468SM, Mheydari2, Gastroking, Shammok, Pineapplelord09, Jnteller15 and Anonymous: 200

- **Ophthalmology in medieval Islam** *Source:* https://en.wikipedia.org/wiki/Ophthalmology_in_medieval_Islam?oldid=671967784 *Contributors:* William M. Connolley, Charles Matthews, Hadal, Kwamikagami, Flammifer, Famousdog, Mdd, Zereshk, Woohookitty, Merlinme, Ruud Koot, Jeff3000, Farhansher, Rjwilmsi, Yuber, AED, Dialectric, Igiffin, SmackBot, Jagged 85, Cplakidas, MrPMonday, Mukadderat, Tktktk, Alice Mudgarden, Hemlock Martinis, Cydebot, Missvain, Nick Number, Dsp13, CommonsDelinker, Nono64, J8079s, Al-Andalusi, Addbot, Tsange, Lightbot, AnomieBOT, Radbod~enwiki, Citation bot 1, EmausBot, John of Reading, Syncategoremata, Aquib American Muslim, Someone65, ClueBot NG, Helpful Pixie Bot, Mughal Lohar, Glacialfox, Skr15081997 and Anonymous: 14

- **Plague doctor costume** *Source:* https://en.wikipedia.org/wiki/Plague_doctor_costume?oldid=690664121 *Contributors:* Shyamal, Xanzzibar, Pretzelpaws, Orpheus, Discospinster, Wareh, BDD, Michael Gäbler, Joygerhardt, Nightscream, Kolbasz, Bloodofox, Kortoso, Nikkimaria, BorgQueen, Akrabbim, SmackBot, McGeddon, Nbarth, Parrot of Doom, Ian Spackman, Mon Vier, Calrion, Oreo Priest, Doug Coldwell, Nev1, Andrewaskew, CMBJ, Flyer22 Reborn, Ngebendi, XLinkBot, Stickee, Good Olfactory, Addbot, Luckas-bot, Yobot, Fraggle81, AnomieBOT, Archon 2488, The High Fin Sperm Whale, LilHelpa, Tyrol5, Mjasfca, Celuici, FrescoBot, Pinethicket, SkyMachine, Anneyh, DARTH SIDIOUS 2, EmausBot, John of Reading, Mashaunix, SidoniaBorcke, ZéroBot, Netha Hussain, ClueBot NG, Jack Greenmaven, MelbourneStar, Hjt1126, Marechal Ney, Costesseyboy, Helpful Pixie Bot, DBigXray, Mitchitara, ChrisGualtieri, Lugia2453, Alderpax, Gajarion27, GampsCrawford, Asdklf;, KH-1, Zackattack1936, Kaysynandliv, Flangis and Anonymous: 60

- **Prophetic medicine** *Source:* https://en.wikipedia.org/wiki/Prophetic_medicine?oldid=685540809 *Contributors:* William M. Connolley, Mpa-tel, Rjwilmsi, DVdm, CambridgeBayWeather, SmackBot, Skizzik, SMasters, Slasher-fun, Seaphoto, Al-Andalusi, Editor2020, Addbot, Yobot, Kwiki, GoingBatty, Rebella123, ClueBot NG, Dr. Persi, Muhamadoqaili, Helpful Pixie Bot, Marcocapelle, BattyBot, HDSKhan, Monkbot and Anonymous: 11

- **Psychology in medieval Islam** *Source:* https://en.wikipedia.org/wiki/Psychology_in_medieval_Islam?oldid=690557878 *Contributors:* William M. Connolley, TimR, Alan Liefting, MisfitToys, Mike Rosoft, YUL89YYZ, Kwamikagami, Famousdog, Woohookitty, Prashanthns, BD2412, Rjwilmsi, Koavf, Todd Vierling, Dialectric, Trovatore, JTBurman, Ragesoss, Reyk, BorgQueen, Palapa, SmackBot, Jagged 85, Delldot, Aeternus, FairuseBot, Eastlaw, Neelix, Hemlock Martinis, Mattisse, Mojo Hand, DuncanHill, Taksen, Dragonnas, Rich257, Gun Powder Ma, R'n'B, CommonsDelinker, Nono64, Adavidb, Belovedfreak, TXiKiBoT, Xe7al, Explicit, ImageRemovalBot, Witchwooder, J8079s, Cirt, Al-Andalusi, Thingg, Xiquet, ZooFari, Addbot, Freud2008, Redheylin, Tassedethe, Lightbot, Yobot, AnomieBOT, Citation bot, Eumolpo, J04n, Citation bot 1, Sahar N Saleem, RjwilmsiBot, EmausBot, John of Reading, Syncategoremata, Aquib American Muslim, Thywob, Someone65, Helpful Pixie Bot, Calabe1992, BG19bot, Mogism, Bruce526, DrRNC, Sharif uddin and Anonymous: 20

4.2 Images

- **File:13th_century_anatomical_illustration_-_sharp.jpg** *Source:* https://upload.wikimedia.org/wikipedia/commons/1/12/13th_century_anatomical_illustration_-_sharp.jpg *License:* Public domain *Contributors:* Bodley library *Original artist:* Anonymous

- **File:A_Sydney_butchers,_1900_(3100789785).jpg** *Source:* https://upload.wikimedia.org/wikipedia/commons/c/c8/A_Sydney_butchers%2C_1900_%283100789785%29.jpg *License:* CC BY 2.0 *Contributors:* A Sydney butcher's, 1900 *Original artist:* Photographic Collection from Australia

- **File:Acral_gangrene_due_to_plague.jpg** *Source:* https://upload.wikimedia.org/wikipedia/commons/8/88/Acral_gangrene_due_to_plague.jpg *License:* Public domain *Contributors:* This media comes from the Centers for Disease Control and Prevention's Public Health Image Library (PHIL), with identification number **#1957**. *Original artist:*

- Original uploaderL M123 at en.wikipedia

- **File:Acral_necrosis_due_to_bubonic_plague.jpg** *Source:* https://upload.wikimedia.org/wikipedia/commons/0/0a/Acral_necrosis_due_to_bubonic_plague.jpg *License:* Public domain *Contributors:* http://emedicine.medscape.com/article/967495-overview *Original artist:* Textbook of Military Medicine. Washington, DC, US Department of the Army, Office of the Surgeon General, and Borden Institute. 1997:493. Government publication, no copyright on photos.

- **File:Al-Risalah_al-Dhahabiah.JPG** *Source:* https://upload.wikimedia.org/wikipedia/commons/b/b3/Al-Risalah_al-Dhahabiah.JPG *License:* CC BY-SA 4.0 *Contributors:* Own work *Original artist:* Thaghalein

- **File:Allah-green.svg** *Source:* https://upload.wikimedia.org/wikipedia/commons/4/4e/Allah-green.svg *License:* Public domain *Contributors:* Converted to SVG from Image:Islam.png, originally from en:Image:Ift32.gif, uploaded to the English Wikipedia by Mr100percent on 4 February 2003. Originally described as "Copied from Public Domain artwork". *Original artist:* ?

- **File:Ambox_important.svg** *Source:* https://upload.wikimedia.org/wikipedia/commons/b/b4/Ambox_important.svg *License:* Public domain *Contributors:* Own work, based off of Image:Ambox scales.svg *Original artist:* Dsmurat (talk · contribs)

- **File:Anatomical_Man.jpg** *Source:* https://upload.wikimedia.org/wikipedia/commons/7/76/Anatomical_Man.jpg *License:* Public domain *Contributors:* Own work *Original artist:* Limbourg brothers

- **File:Anthrax_PHIL_2033.png** *Source:* https://upload.wikimedia.org/wikipedia/commons/5/5f/Anthrax_PHIL_2033.png *License:* Public domain *Contributors:* This media comes from the Centers for Disease Control and Prevention's Public Health Image Library (PHIL), with identification number **#2033**. *Original artist:* CDC/ James H. Steele

- **File:Beak_doctor_mask.jpg** *Source:* https://upload.wikimedia.org/wikipedia/commons/8/8c/Beak_doctor_mask.jpg *License:* CC BY 2.0 *Contributors:* http://www.flickr.com/photos/tracyelaine/3264042469/ *Original artist:* Flickr: Tracy

- **File:Blackdeath2.gif** *Source:* https://upload.wikimedia.org/wikipedia/commons/d/d3/Blackdeath2.gif *License:* Public domain *Contributors:* Created by the author *Original artist:* The original uploader was Andrei nacu at English Wikipedia

- **File:Bubonic_plague_victims-mass_grave_in_Martigues,_France_1720-1721.jpg** *Source:* https://upload.wikimedia.org/wikipedia/commons/1/1b/Bubonic_plague_victims-mass_grave_in_Martigues%2C_France_1720-1721.jpg *License:* Public domain *Contributors:* http://wwwnc.cdc.gov/eid/article/13/2/06-0197-f1.htm *Original artist:* S. Tzortzis

- **File:Burying_Plague_Victims_of_Tournai.jpg** *Source:* https://upload.wikimedia.org/wikipedia/commons/7/7d/Burying_Plague_Victims_of_Tournai.jpg *License:* Public domain *Contributors:* http://supotnitskiy.ru/stat/stat8.htm *Original artist:* Unknown

- **File:COLLECTIE_TROPENMUSEUM_Karolanden._Huis_van_den_beheerder_van_het_lepra_asyl_te_Lau_Simomo_TMnr_10016893.jpg** *Source:* https://upload.wikimedia.org/wikipedia/commons/e/e2/COLLECTIE_TROPENMUSEUM_Karolanden._Huis_van_den_beheerder_van_het_lepra_asyl_te_Lau_Simomo_TMnr_10016893.jpg *License:* CC BY-SA 3.0 *Contributors:* Tropenmuseum <a href='//commons.wikimedia.org/wiki/Institution:Tropenmuseum' title='Link back to Institution infobox template'><img alt='Link back to Institution infobox template' src='https://upload.wikimedia.org/wikipedia/commons/thumb/7/73/Blue_pencil.svg/15px-Blue_pencil.svg.png' width='15' height='15' srcset='https://upload.wikimedia.org/wikipedia/commons/thumb/7/73/Blue_pencil.svg/23px-Blue_pencil.svg.png 1.5x, https://upload.wikimedia.org/wikipedia/commons/thumb/7/73/Blue_pencil.svg/30px-Blue_pencil.svg.png 2x' data-file-width='600' data-file-height='600' /></a> <a href='//www.wikidata.org/wiki/Q1131589' title='wikidata:Q1131589'><img alt='wikidata:Q1131589' src='https://upload.wikimedia.org/wikipedia/commons/thumb/f/ff/Wikidata-logo.svg/20px-Wikidata-logo.svg.png' width='20' height='11' srcset='https://upload.wikimedia.org/wikipedia/commons/thumb/f/ff/Wikidata-logo.svg/30px-Wikidata-logo.svg.png 1.5x, https://upload.wikimedia.org/wikipedia/commons/thumb/f/ff/Wikidata-logo.svg/40px-Wikidata-logo.svg.png 2x' data-file-width='1050' data-file-height='590' /></a> *Original artist:* Tassilo Adam

- **File:Canons_of_medicine.JPG** *Source:* https://upload.wikimedia.org/wikipedia/commons/f/f7/Canons_of_medicine.JPG *License:* Public domain *Contributors:* personal picture *Original artist:* en:User:Zereshk

- **File:Chacachacare.JPG** *Source:* https://upload.wikimedia.org/wikipedia/commons/6/68/Chacachacare.JPG *License:* CC-BY-SA-3.0 *Contributors:* ? *Original artist:* ?

- **File:Cheshm_manuscript.jpg** *Source:* https://upload.wikimedia.org/wikipedia/commons/a/a6/Cheshm_manuscript.jpg *License:* Public domain *Contributors:* ? *Original artist:* ?

- **File:Chumbunt.png** *Source:* https://upload.wikimedia.org/wikipedia/commons/7/74/Chumbunt.png *License:* Public domain *Contributors:* ? *Original artist:* ?

- **File:Commons-logo.svg** *Source:* https://upload.wikimedia.org/wikipedia/en/4/4a/Commons-logo.svg *License:* ? *Contributors:* ? *Original artist:* ?

- **File:Coronation_Chair_Denmark_(King).jpg** *Source:* https://upload.wikimedia.org/wikipedia/commons/6/68/Coronation_Chair_Denmark_%28King%29.jpg *License:* CC BY-SA 3.0 *Contributors:* This file has been **extracted** from another file: Rosenborg castle 8.jpg. *Original artist:* Sven Rosborn

- **File:Dagger-14-plain.png** *Source:* https://upload.wikimedia.org/wikipedia/commons/3/37/Dagger-14-plain.png *License:* CC0 *Contributors:* Own work *Original artist:* RexxS

- **File:Danse_macabre_by_Michael_Wolgemut.png** *Source:* https://upload.wikimedia.org/wikipedia/commons/b/bf/Danse_macabre_by_Michael_Wolgemut.png *License:* Public domain *Contributors:* ? *Original artist:* ?

- **File:Dent_de_narval.jpg** *Source:* https://upload.wikimedia.org/wikipedia/commons/7/74/Dent_de_narval.jpg *License:* CC BY-SA 3.0 *Contributors:* Own work *Original artist:* Licorne37

- **File:Directions_for_searchers,_Pune_plague_of_1897.jpg** *Source:* https://upload.wikimedia.org/wikipedia/commons/7/75/Directions_for_searchers%2C_Pune_plague_of_1897.jpg *License:* Public domain *Contributors:* This image is available from the **National Library of Scotland**
Original artist: Government Officer, British India.

- **File:Medical_book_front_page.jpg** *Source:* https://upload.wikimedia.org/wikipedia/commons/7/74/Medical_book_front_page.jpg *License:* CC BY-SA 3.0 *Contributors:* Own work *Original artist:* Nannadeem

- **File:Medieval_dentistry.jpg** *Source:* https://upload.wikimedia.org/wikipedia/commons/0/0b/Medieval_dentistry.jpg *License:* Public domain *Contributors:* ? *Original artist:* ?

- **File:Merge-arrow.svg** *Source:* https://upload.wikimedia.org/wikipedia/commons/a/aa/Merge-arrow.svg *License:* Public domain *Contributors:* ? *Original artist:* ?

- **File:Mondino_-_Anathomia,_1541_-_3022668.tif** *Source:* https://upload.wikimedia.org/wikipedia/commons/1/1c/Mondino_-_Anathomia%2C_1541_-_3022668.tif *License:* Public domain *Contributors:* Available in the digital library of the European Library of Information and Culture and uploaded in partnership (ID: '). *Original artist:* Mondino : dei Liucci

- **File:Naskh_script_-_Qur'anic_verses.jpg** *Source:* https://upload.wikimedia.org/wikipedia/commons/0/05/Naskh_script_-_Qur%27anic_verses.jpg *License:* Public domain *Contributors:* Library of Congress *Original artist:* Unknown Calligrapher

- **File:Paul_Fürst,_Der_Doctor_Schnabel_von_Rom_(Holländer_version).png** *Source:* https://upload.wikimedia.org/wikipedia/commons/5/57/Paul_F%C3%BCrst%2C_Der_Doctor_Schnabel_von_Rom_%28Holl%C3%A4nder_version%29.png *License:* Public domain *Contributors:* Internet Archive's copy of Eugen Holländer, *Original artist:* I. Columbina, ad vivum delineavit. Paulus Fürst Excud[i]t. I [or J] Columbina has not, I think, been identified. Paul Fürst (1608–1666) was the publisher, and perhaps also the engraver.

- **File:Plague_bubo.jpg** *Source:* https://upload.wikimedia.org/wikipedia/commons/5/5e/Plague_bubo.jpg *License:* Public domain *Contributors:* http://www.cdc.gov/NCIDOD/DVBID/plague/diagnosis.htm *Original artist:* U.S. Center for Disease Control

- **File:Question_book-new.svg** *Source:* https://upload.wikimedia.org/wikipedia/en/9/99/Question_book-new.svg *License:* Cc-by-sa-3.0 *Contributors:*
  Created from scratch in Adobe Illustrator. Based on Image:Question book.png created by User:Equazcion *Original artist:*
  Tkgd2007

- **File:Rod_of_Asclepius2.svg** *Source:* https://upload.wikimedia.org/wikipedia/commons/e/e3/Rod_of_Asclepius2.svg *License:* CC BY-SA 3.0 *Contributors:* This file was derived from: Rod of asclepius.png
  Original artist:

- Original: CatherinMunro

- **File:Spinalonga.jpeg** *Source:* https://upload.wikimedia.org/wikipedia/commons/b/b6/Spinalonga.jpeg *License:* Public domain *Contributors:* No machine-readable source provided. Own work assumed (based on copyright claims). *Original artist:* No machine-readable author provided. Malamant~commonswiki assumed (based on copyright claims).

- **File:The_Metropolitan_M_Stamp.PNG** *Source:* https://upload.wikimedia.org/wikipedia/commons/c/c0/The_Metropolitan_M_Stamp.PNG *License:* CC BY-SA 3.0 *Contributors:* Own work *Original artist:* Unisouth

- **File:Thomé_Salix_alba_clean.jpg** *Source:* https://upload.wikimedia.org/wikipedia/commons/a/a1/Thom%C3%A9_Salix_alba_clean.jpg *License:* Public domain *Contributors:* ? *Original artist:* ?

- **File:Trombidium.jpg** *Source:* https://upload.wikimedia.org/wikipedia/commons/0/0c/Trombidium.jpg *License:* CC BY-SA 3.0 *Contributors:* Own work *Original artist:* Pankaj Oudhia

- **File:Unbalanced_scales.svg** *Source:* https://upload.wikimedia.org/wikipedia/commons/f/fe/Unbalanced_scales.svg *License:* Public domain *Contributors:* ? *Original artist:* ?

- **File:ViennaDioscoridesFolio483vBirds.jpg** *Source:* https://upload.wikimedia.org/wikipedia/commons/3/34/ViennaDioscoridesFolio483vBirds.jpg *License:* Public domain *Contributors:* ? *Original artist:* ?

- **File:Weltliche_Schatzkammer_Wienb.jpg** *Source:* https://upload.wikimedia.org/wikipedia/commons/8/8a/Weltliche_Schatzkammer_Wienb.jpg *License:* Public domain *Contributors:* Own work *Original artist:* MyName (Gryffindor) stitched by Marku1988

- **File:Wiki_letter_w.svg** *Source:* https://upload.wikimedia.org/wikipedia/en/6/6c/Wiki_letter_w.svg *License:* Cc-by-sa-3.0 *Contributors:* ? *Original artist:* ?

- **File:Wiki_letter_w_cropped.svg** *Source:* https://upload.wikimedia.org/wikipedia/commons/1/1c/Wiki_letter_w_cropped.svg *License:* CC-BY-SA-3.0 *Contributors:*

- Wiki_letter_w.svg *Original artist:* Wiki_letter_w.svg: Jarkko Piiroinen

- **File:Wikibooks-logo-en-noslogan.svg** *Source:* https://upload.wikimedia.org/wikipedia/commons/d/df/Wikibooks-logo-en-noslogan.svg *License:* CC BY-SA 3.0 *Contributors:* Own work *Original artist:* User:Bastique, User:Ramac et al.

- **File:Wikiquote-logo.svg** *Source:* https://upload.wikimedia.org/wikipedia/commons/f/fa/Wikiquote-logo.svg *License:* Public domain *Contributors:* ? *Original artist:* ?

- **File:Wikiversity-logo.svg** *Source:* https://upload.wikimedia.org/wikipedia/commons/9/91/Wikiversity-logo.svg *License:* CC BY-SA 3.0 *Contributors:* Snorky (optimized and cleaned up by verdy_p) *Original artist:* Snorky (optimized and cleaned up by verdy_p)

- **File:World_distribution_of_plague_1998.PNG** *Source:* https://upload.wikimedia.org/wikipedia/commons/6/6b/World_distribution_of_plague_1998.PNG *License:* Public domain *Contributors:* ? *Original artist:* ?

- **File:Xenopsylla_chepsis_(oriental_rat_flea).jpg** *Source:* https://upload.wikimedia.org/wikipedia/commons/2/25/Xenopsylla_chepsis_%28oriental_rat_flea%29.jpg *License:* Public domain *Contributors:* http://www.cdc.gov/ncidod/dvbid/plague/cheob6x4.htm *Original artist:* Centers for Disease Control and Prevention

- **File:Yersinia_pestis_fluorescent.jpeg** *Source:* https://upload.wikimedia.org/wikipedia/commons/1/15/Yersinia_pestis_fluorescent.jpeg *License:* Public domain *Contributors:* Transferred from en.wikipedia to Commons by Fvasconcellos. *Original artist:*

  - Photo Credit=

  - Content Providers= CDC/ Courtesy of Larry Stauffer, Oregon State Public Health Laboratory

4.3   Content license